Mental Health in Pregnancy and Childbirth

For Elsevier:

Commissioning Editor: Mary Seager/Mairi McCubbin
Development Editor: Rebecca Nelemans
Project Manager: Joannah Duncan
Designer: Andy Chapman

Mental Health in Pregnancy and Childbirth

Edited by

Sally Price BSc(Hons) MSc PGCertEd RM MICG NNEB

Consultant Midwife, North Bristol NHS Trust and the University of the West of
England, Bristol, UK

CHURCHILL
LIVINGSTONE

ELSEVIER

EDINBURGH LONDON NEW YORK OXFORD PHILADELPHIA ST LOUIS SYDNEY TORONTO 2007

CHURCHILL
LIVINGSTONE
ELSEVIER

© 2007, Elsevier Limited. All rights reserved.

No part of this publication may be reproduced, stored in a retrieval system, or
transmitted in any form or by any means, electronic, mechanical, photocopying,
recording or otherwise, without the prior permission of the Publishers.
Permissions may be sought directly from Elsevier's Health Sciences Rights
Department, 1600 John F. Kennedy Boulevard, Suite 1800, Philadelphia, PA
19103-2899, USA: phone: (+1) 215 239 3804; fax: (+1) 215 239 3805; or, e-mail:
healthpermissions@elsevier.com. You may also complete your request on-line via
the Elsevier homepage (http://www.elsevier.com), by selecting 'Support and
contact' and then 'Copyright and Permission'.

First published 2007

ISBN-10: 0 443 10317 8

ISBN-13: 978 0 443 10317 9

British Library Cataloguing in Publication Data
A catalogue record for this book is available from the British Library

Library of Congress Cataloging in Publication Data
A catalog record for this book is available from the Library of Congress

Knowledge and best practice in this field are constantly changing. As new
research and experience broaden our knowledge, changes in practice, treatment
and drug therapy may become necessary or appropriate. Readers are advised
to check the most current information provided (i) on procedures featured
or (ii) by the manufacturer of each product to be administered, to verify the
recommended dose or formula, the method and duration of administration, and
contraindications. It is the responsibility of the practitioner, relying on their own
experience and knowledge of the patient, to make diagnoses, to determine
dosages and the best treatment for each individual patient, and to take all
appropriate safety precautions. To the fullest extent of the law, neither the
publisher nor the editors assumes any liability for any injury and/or damage.

The Publisher

ELSEVIER your source for books,
journals and multimedia
in the health sciences
www.elsevierhealth.com

Working together to grow
libraries in developing countries
www.elsevier.com | www.bookaid.org | www.sabre.org

ELSEVIER BOOK AID International Sabre Foundation

The
publisher's
policy is to use
paper manufactured
from sustainable forests

Printed in China

Contents

Contributors

Kathleen Marion Baird BSc(Hons) MA (Ed) PGDipHE RM HDE
Senior Midwifery Lecturer, University of the West of England, Bristol, UK

Victoria Blunsden BSc(Hons) RMDip CertEd RN
Specialist Midwife, North Bristol NHS Trust, Bristol, UK

Kathryn Gutteridge MSc PGDip SEN RGN RM
Consultant Midwife, University Hospitals of Leicester NHS Trust, Leicester, UK
Psychotherapist, Private Practice, UK

Peter Hadwin BSc(Hons) MSc PGCE CertCAT RMN
Senior Lecturer, University of the West of England, Bristol, UK
Counsellor, Primary Care, UK
Psychotherapist, Private Practice, UK

Jennifer Hall MSc PGDip(HE) RN RM ADM
Senior Midwifery Lecturer, University of the West of England, Bristol, UK

Anthony Harrison MSc DipN RMN
Consultant Nurse (Liaison Psychiatry), Avon & Wiltshire Mental Health Partnership NHS Trust, UK
Visiting Research Fellow, Faculty of Health and Social Care, University of the West of England, Bristol, UK

Victoria Lavender BA(Hons) MA(Phil) CertEd RMN
Senior Lecturer, School of Mental Health and Learning Disabilities, University of the West of England, Bristol, UK

Rosemary Mander MSc PhD RGN SCM MTD
Professor of Midwifery, University of Edinburgh, Edinburgh, UK

Sian Monahan PDCHyp RMN MBSCH
Clinical Nurse Specialist, Bristol Specialist Drug Service, Bristol, UK

Sally Price BSc(Hons) MSc PGCertEd RM MICG NNEB
Consultant Midwife, North Bristol NHS Trust and the University of the West of England, Bristol, UK

Nigel Philip Weeks MA CertEd(FE) RMN RCNT
Senior Lecturer, Mental Health Nursing, University of the West of England, Bristol, UK

Stephanie Withers BSc(Hons) RN RM ONC
Delivery Suite Manager, North Bristol NHS Trust, Bristol, UK

Preface

Mental illness is a leading cause of maternal death (NICE 2004). Women with mental health disorders are also subject to stereotyping and prejudice in their interactions with health services. Midwives may find providing care for women with mental health problems challenging. Indeed the evidence would suggest that this is an area where midwives need to improve their knowledge and understanding (Stewart & Henshaw 2002). Currently women with mental health problems cannot be guaranteed maternity care that understands or meets their needs. The midwifery profession and related disciplines generally require an improved awareness of common mental health problems, how they relate to pregnancy and what they can do professionally and personally to help. There is also a need to dispel the stigma associated with mental illness and promote sensitive, evidence-based, woman-centred care. Unfortunately, the current professional literature base reflects the minimisation of this topic within the dominant discourse, and midwives and others are without guidance or support for their practice.

The aim of this book is to inform and influence midwifery practice and those who have contact with pregnant women, to support those who have mental health problems. It has been written by a combination of practising experts in the fields of both midwifery and mental health. The text includes information on some of the more common mental health disorders and explores their relationship with pregnancy. Mechanisms that can be adopted to promote mental health are addressed, including statutory services, alternative and complimentary therapies, web-based resources, and voluntary organisations as well as clinical healthcare interventions. Hopefully, by reflecting on the content of this book, health professionals will carefully consider their care approach to women with mental health problems, promoting a positive experience of a fair and effective maternity service.

Bristol, 2007   Sally Price

References

National Institute for Clinical Excellence, The Scottish Executive Health Department and The Department of Health Social Services and Public Safety: Northern Ireland 2004 The confidential enquires into maternal deaths in the United Kingdom. Why mothers die 2000–2002. RCOG, London

Stewart C, Henshaw C 2002 Midwives and perinatal mental health. British Journal of Midwifery 10(2):117–121

Chapter **1**

Learning from women's experience of mental illness

Sally Price

INTRODUCTION

Many women in the UK will experience mental health problems. Although this is also true of men, there are significant differences in the way that mental illness occurs in women and men, and how mental illness impacts on their lives. Anxiety, depression and eating disorders are more common in women, with substance misuse and antisocial personality disorders more common in men (Gold 1998). However, physiological differences such as pregnancy and birth may increase women's risk of mental illness. Women are also more likely to experience somatic illness as a result of their psychological problems. However, women's mental health should not be defined by their biology, but through the context of their lives, their powerlessness and lack of social status and experiences of violence and abuse (Department of Health, DoH 2002a). Women are more likely than men to experience health inequalities that cause or compound mental illness, such as poverty and lone parenting. Certain groups of women such as those from black and minority ethnic groups, lesbian and bisexual women and women offenders are more vulnerable to mental health problems. The impact of the low value placed on women's work by society may also have a negative impact on self-esteem and contribute to women's mental illness.

This chapter will consider why mental healthcare is relevant to maternity care and the professional practice of midwives and others who work within the maternity services. It will also highlight the importance of listening to service users and learning from their experiences.

Promoting mental health has been identified as a core standard for healthcare within the National Service Framework for Mental

Health. An important part of this standard is combating discrimi-nation against individuals and groups with mental health problems and promoting their social inclusion (DoH 1999a). Yet, little attention appears to be paid to promoting mental health within midwifery practice. Combined with this, scant attention is paid to women with pre-existing mental illness or the impact their preg-nancy may have on them and their mental health. This leads to an assumption that perhaps the maternity services are not listening to the women they serve, particularly in relation to mental health. Few studies exploring the perspective of women service users exist, but there is some evidence that 'women express an overwhelming sense of not being listened to, that their life experiences, views and needs are not validated or responded to' (DoH 2002a). With this in mind, it seems obvious that midwives must be willing and able to listen to the woman's views about her care needs.

LISTENING TO WOMEN

Women who experience a mental illness such as obsessive–compulsive disorder (OCD) may find pregnancy and birth worsens their illness.

One of the most important things that health professionals can do is to validate and learn from women's experience of mental illness by listening to their stories and their views. One woman tells her story of what it was like for her to experience OCD during her first pregnancy.

'To me the whole of my pregnancy was a tremendous risk. Soon after I found out I was pregnant OCD began to take hold. Initially I was worried about having a child with Down's syndrome, and then I became worried about catching toxoplasmosis from our pet cats. Taking tests to reassure myself had little effect. I would think – what if the test result was wrong? How can they be 100% accurate? Doubts crept into my mind paralysing me with anxiety.

Very soon, I was viewing everyday activities as huge contamination risks. For example, the washing-up would meticulously be washed, then washed and re-washed, because in my mind it may have touched the floor or the cats may have touched it. Although I knew rationally that this was not the case, the persistent thoughts told me I might have done it and that chance was a risk I could not take. I had to be absolutely sure I wasn't contaminating myself and therefore the baby. My whole day and every waking moment of the night (of which there were many) became full of intrusive, anxiety provoking thoughts, which placed me in a state of permanent panic.

I could not eat my breakfast, for fear cat litter (more specifically faeces) may have got in it. I would make two or three bowls of cereal throwing each away for fear it was contaminated. Eventually I would give up and go without breakfast because I felt not eating was a safer option than eating and contaminating or poisoning my baby.

I became a prisoner in my own house. I was so phobic about the cats, because of my fear of toxoplasmosis; I would try and live in one room, staying away from them. However, this did not stop the anxiety, because on occasions when I had to walk past the cat litter tray I would think I could have eaten cat faeces. These thoughts filled me with disgust, but they were very real. Eventually I decided it would be easier if I stayed out of the house all day, in an effort to make my life more bearable.

So each morning I would wash and re-wash myself in the bath, taking as long as an hour. My husband would have to watch me wash my face and clean my teeth, in order to ensure I wasn't taking any bathroom chemicals into my mouth. I would find myself repeating complex rituals, involving repetition of washing and frequently spitting into the sink, just in case, despite my husband watching, I had taken any chemicals into my mouth. After this, my husband would make my breakfast and watch me eat it, because I was frightened I might put kitchen chemicals or cat faeces into my breakfast bowl. I was clearly terrified of harming my baby in some way, and my OCD thoughts and rituals were concerned with protecting the baby from any harm.

When my husband left the house, so did I. I would drive around until a shopping centre opened. Even driving around in my car I felt I could drink the petrol. By being in a place where lots of others people were, I felt slightly reassured, because I reasoned if I was behaving in a bizarre way, for example touching the floor, bins or dog faeces on the pavement, people would stare at me. Likewise, the only way I could get myself to eat was in a public restaurant. This way I believed people would stare if I tried to contaminate my food in any way. Even then I was restricted in the foods I could eat because of my anxiety and always used a knife and fork. I felt it was too great a risk to use my hands to handle food as they may have been contaminated.

Toilet visits were another ordeal. I would inspect toilet after toilet for cleanliness, then when using the toilet be anxious of touching anything I considered contaminated. There would follow a ritual of hand washing that was repeated many times. Because the excessive washing was embarrassing when people were around, I would return a few minutes later to wash again once they had gone.

After spending hours in the shopping centre, I would return home and stay in one room until my husband returned home. At this point, he would watch me eat and wash my hands to reassure me that I wasn't contaminating myself. Despite his reassurances I was forever asking him questions such as "are you sure those vegetables are properly washed?", consequently doubting his judgement too. This obviously put a tremendous strain on my husband and our relationship, and I was very grateful for his patience and support. The whole duration of my pregnancy was a living nightmare for me, and an incredible stress on my husband. This is so typical of OCD, which affects the whole family because its effects are so very debilitating. Thankfully there was light at the end of the tunnel – but only after the baby was born and years of cognitive behavioural therapy, combined with drug treatment'.

This woman's experience has highlighted how traumatic suffering from OCD in pregnancy can be. By telling her story she hopes that others will be able to find the help and support that they so desperately need from those involved with her maternity care. To do this effectively, health professionals should understand and appreciate the impact of a mental health disorder on the woman and her pregnancy. For example OCD is often kept a secret by the sufferer, so it is important health professionals encourage women to talk about any anxieties. They should also be aware of any symptoms of OCD, such as high anxiety, preoccupation and depression. It is imperative that they can empathise with women, and help them to identify their changing needs in light of the pregnancy. Midwives may be able to point women in the direction of appropriate services, particularly those that provide listening and talking or complimentary therapies, along with the development of coping skills and strategies.

There are complex problems associated with meeting the mental healthcare needs of pregnant women, for example, the need to balance the benefits of continued psychiatric drug treatments during pregnancy where the effects on the fetus may be harmful or unknown. A multi-disciplinary approach is essential if both maternity and psychiatric needs are to be met. The role of the midwife must be to act as an advocate for the women and ensure her needs are fully addressed. To be an effective advocate, midwives should act as a vehicle to convey their client's perspective to others. This means interpreting or representing the client's needs and views, arguing those views and needs and supporting clients to represent themselves to others. To do this effectively, practitioners need to develop skills of negotiation, empathy and assertiveness (Hart 2004).

However, women who seek help may be unable to access appropriate care or be expected to fit into services commonly used by and designed for men. They may feel threatened or vulnerable in a mixed sex therapeutic environment, particularly if they have previous experiences of violence or abuse. An inconsistency and lack of coordinated services have also been identified as major factors in perinatal mental healthcare (Church & Scanlan 2002). The lack of psychiatric mother and baby units may mean the woman is separated from her baby in order to receive the care she needs. Not only is there a lack of specialist facilities for postnatal women with mental illness, but being pregnant may exclude women from mainstream high dependency psychiatric services. The acutely ill pregnant or postnatal woman is therefore left without the specialist care she needs. Given this lack of services to meet women's needs, it is hardly surprising that suicide is a leading cause of maternal death (National Institute for Clinical Excellence, NICE 2004).

A PUBLIC HEALTH ISSUE

Suicide is a national public health issue. The need to reduce deaths from suicide has been identified with a target reduction of 20% by 2010 (DoH 1999b). A national suicide prevention strategy has been formulated with several goals, including reducing the risk of suicide in high-risk groups and promoting mental well-being in the wider population (DoH 2002b). Midwives clearly have a role within this strategy, with suicide the cause of the majority of maternal deaths reported to the Confidential Enquiries into Maternal Deaths within the triennium of 2000–2002 (NICE 2004). However, problems with reporting maternal deaths from suicide have been identified, with many more actual cases likely. Risk factors for perinatal mental health problems have also been identified, such as previous serious mental illness. As a result of this, recommendations have been made that midwives should enquire about the woman's psychiatric history at booking (NICE et al 2001). However, research has identified that few midwives have had specialist training in this field and many would require further support before taking on this role (Stewart & Henshaw 2002).

Bloom (2001) highlights the delicate balance between professional responsibility, the client's wishes and the availability of psychological therapies. Without professional development opportunities and an understanding of the availability and role of local mental health services, it may be difficult for midwives to achieve this balance. However, despite these challenges midwives are in an ideal position to identify mental health problems among the women they work with. An example of good practice is the Brierley Midwifery Practice, who have identified how women with mental health problems often have little stability in their lives, and that continuity of care may help clients to develop trusting relationships with midwives. This also leads to the midwife knowing the woman and thus being in a better position to identify behavioural changes and expedite referrals to support services (Douglas & Arias 2001).

CONCLUSION

It is essential that midwives recognise, accept and address the causes of women's mental illness and their mental health needs if they are to provide holistic women-centred maternity care. One way to achieve this is by truly listening to women and their families about their experiences, life challenges and how their health is affected. Considering service user perspectives in relation to mental health will only serve to enhance both individualised care and the maternity services as a whole.

References

Bloom J 2001 Midwifery and perinatal mental health provision. British Journal of Midwifery 9:385–388

Church S, Scanlan M 2002 Meeting the needs of women with mental health problems. Practical Midwife 5:10–12

Department of Health (DoH) 1999a National service framework for mental health. Department of Health, London

Department of Health (DoH) 1999b Saving lives: our healthier nation. Department of Health, London

Department of Health (DoH) 2002a Women's mental health: into the mainstream. Strategic development of mental health care for women. Department of Health, London

Department of Health (DoH) 2002b National suicide prevention strategy for England. Department of Health, London

Douglas J, Arias T 2001 Mental health. Midwives in action: a resource. English National Board for Nursing Midwifery and Health Visiting, London

Gold J 1998 Gender differences in psychiatric illness and treatments: a critical review. Journal of Nervous and Mental Disease 186:769–775

Hart D 2004 The recognition of inequality and the need for empowerment. In: Kirby S, Hart D, Cross D et al (eds) Mental health nursing. Competencies for practice. Palgrave MacMillan, Basingstoke, p 13–31

National Institute for Clinical Excellence (NICE) 2004, (funded by The Scottish Executive Health Department and The Department of Health Social Services and Public Safety: Northern Ireland) The confidential enquires into maternal deaths in the United Kingdom. Why mothers die 2000–2002. RCOG Press, London

National Institute for Clinical Excellence (NICE), The Scottish Executive Health Department and The Department of Health Social Services and Public Safety: Northern Ireland 2001 The confidential enquiries into maternal deaths in the United Kingdom. Why mothers die 1997–1999. RCOG Press, London

Stewart C, Henshaw C 2002 Midwives and perinatal mental health. British Journal of Midwifery 10:117–121

Chapter 2

Understanding mental health: theoretical approaches

Kathryn Gutteridge

INTRODUCTION

The century in which we live prides itself on tolerance, acceptance and development of the 'self'. However, if someone is suffering from a mental illness or displays eccentric behaviour, then our society is less tolerant and empathic than we would like to believe. Understanding how we think and therefore behave is important and gives insight into the innermost intricacies of the human psyche. Being in possession of this information enables health professionals to achieve a deeper knowledge of the person seeking care in clinical situations. This chapter will discuss the theoretical models applied to mental health and illness, including biological, sociological and psychological perspectives and consider some contemporary approaches to treatment.

A BIOMEDICAL UNDERSTANDING OF MENTAL ILLNESS

Biomedicine is based upon the assumption that disease is an organic condition and dispels non-organic factors associated with emotional behaviours and symptoms. Thus, the patient is seen as a recipient of disease, separate from any other factor and is best treated in hospital where investigation and treatment can be controlled, a scientific or positivist process.

Disease categorisation was first established in the sixteenth century and later extended into more general use by the physician William Cullen, published in 1785 under the title *Synopsis Nosologiae Methodical* (University of Virginia Health System 1998). Cullen coined the phrase 'neurosis'. His theories claimed that disease was the result of disturbances of the nervous system. Modern day

Table 2.1 The Diagnostic and Statistical Manual of Mental Disorders IV

Axis I	Clinical syndromes and other conditions that may be a focus of clinical attention
	All mental disorders except personality disorders and mental retardation
Axis II	Personality disorders
	Life-long deeply ingrained inflexible and maladaptive behaviours, likely to affect an individual's ability to be treated
Axis III	General medical conditions
	Any condition that might affect an individual's mental state and be relevant to treatment
Axis IV	Psychosocial and environmental problems
	Events such as divorce, bereavement or other life events, ratings are made and scored from 1–7. 7 is considered catastrophic
Axis V	Global assessment of functioning
	Psychosocial, social and occupational functioning. 0 equal to persistent danger and 100 equates to superior functioning

(American Psychiatric Association 1991)

understanding of mental illness and models of psychiatry fit this descriptor. Symptoms are categorised and given a diagnosis or label enabling treatments to be formulated. The World Health Organization produced an organised classification of mental disorders in the International Classification of Diseases-6 (ICD-6) published in 1948, and in 1952 the American Psychiatric Association published *The Diagnostic and Statistical Manual of Mental Disorders* (DSM-I) identifying 106 diagnostic categories (Table 2.1).

Biomedical approaches to mental illness view the problem through abnormal biophysiological functioning. This approach puts genetic and biochemical factors in the frame. Examples of this would be:

● Depression: caused by a dysfunction of neuronal transmission and a biochemical reduction in serotonin uptake
● Schizophrenia: a genetic-inherited deficiency producing schizoid symptoms and behaviours.

Both of these conditions are explained using a reductionalist approach in terms of object physiology and biochemistry. While successful in the identification and treatment of organic disease this approach is skewed in terms of understanding mental illness.

Describing behaviour as abnormal is precarious. Human behaviour is complex and it is perhaps impossible to apply value judgements that are rooted within a unique cultural context. This view is explored by Thomas Szasz (1994), who describes mental illness as a 'metaphorical illness' since the mind is not an organ and cannot be subjected to examination in the same way as other organic structures. Ronald Laing (1967), famous for his anti-psychiatry views, campaigned against dehumanisation of the patient. He formed the opinion that medication had a value but sought to include the mentally ill in humankind rather than in secure asylums.

Evidence that biomedicine has sought to control mentally ill women is referred to as far back as the Middle Ages, when women were accused of stirring men's passions and seen as agents of the devil. The unpredictability of women's reproductive cycle and hormones make them vulnerable to the biomedical approach, since it challenges the scientific male ego (Doyal 1995). There is also contemporary reference to biomedical factors as a cause of mental illness. Women's susceptibility to developing mental illness is thought to be increased because of the way the sexes develop, with serotonin being produced in greater quantities in men than women (Nishizawa et al 1997).

The dominant discourse of mental illness over the last century expresses discontent with the biomedical model and consequently has supported the dissolution of large psychiatric institutions. The culture of medical dominance has been challenged and a reconsideration of a social understanding of mental health proposed with a return to community care (Mora 1980). Today modern thinking acknowledges biomedicine as a persuasive model but since mental illness is not wholly scientifically determined it may be better understood within an integrative framework.

THE SOCIAL CONSTRUCTION OF MENTAL ILLNESS

Mental illness has to some extent an uneasy relationship with sociology. Many notable sociological theories are in conflict with the positivist constructs of modern psychiatric medicine. A social construction of mental illness seeks to understand the individual in the perspective of their life; considering how systems and structures influence and impact upon the professional in all situations.

There are five main theoretical approaches to health and sociology:

1. Parsonsian functionalism
2. Symbolic interactionism
3. Marxist theory
4. Feminist theory
5. Foucaldian theory.

Parsonsian functionalism

This sociological theory views the role of sick people and their impact upon society (Parsons 1951). The 'sick role' is identified as a legitimate function and to some degree an occupation requiring support, care and treatment through accessing professional systems.

Parsons coined the term 'sick role' in the 1950s, when he drew attention to an individual's motivation into adopting illness and seeking treatment. When ill, it is normal for the sick person to withdraw from society, and be subsumed by services for the unwell. Parsons called this behaviour deviance, and thus the individual feeds the power of the professional by seeking medical treatments and advice. Medical treatments are used to control and reduce symptoms, therefore manipulating the individual out of the sick role and back into societal functioning.

It is possible to argue the robustness of Parsons' theory within a context of mental health, as restoration of normal functioning is always expected but may not be guaranteed. There is an assumption that the sick person will recognise their illness and seek treatment from a professional, and that once in the consultation or undergoing treatment that they will become obedient or compliant.

However, gender-based criticism of Parsons' theory draws attention to medical bias when treating women. Suggesting that some complaints may be termed 'female maladies or neuroses' may result in the misdiagnosis of genuine illnesses (Doyal 1995). This model also fails during pregnancy, which is considered a transitional state of normality for women. Although the pregnant woman seeks advice and occasionally treatment there is no diagnosis of ill health but rather a deviation from the norm.

The sick role is useful, despite criticism, when considering mental health. Waitzkin (1971) drew attention to the fact that some deviance is desirable especially when protecting society against potentially dangerous individuals, with mental hospitals offering a useful function. The theory of the sick role has also drawn attention to the career or occupational status of illness, and many of those who are ill may approach their poor health through this model. However, this career approach is not accessible to those with psychotic diagnoses as they are described as having no control over their mental health. Thus, this theory is found to be lacking in much of the mental health domain.

Symbolic interactionism

Symbolic interactionism describes the interaction between those who are ill and those providing support and care. As a major sociological health theory, the core concept is that illness is a form of social deviance and not necessarily the result of disease. This theory explores the interplay between patient and doctor and how both manipulate situations dependent upon stages of illness – there is a continuum of interactions played out in a metaphorical theatre.

One primary proponent of this theory was Max Weber, a German sociologist, rooted in the notions of the philosopher George Mead. They both described and emphasised the subjective meaning of human behaviour, the social process and pragmatism. However, Herbert Blumer, who studied with Mead, is responsible for coining the term 'symbolic interactionism' (Blumer 1969). This concept allows individuals to understand the world in terms of another's viewpoint, through language, physical environment and symbolism. This suggests that 'the self' is a real construct and created through our own image and a schemata of perceptions that form a dynamic vision of what we are like and what we might like to be.

The representation is elaborated by self-definition and achieved by labelling, such as the name by which we are known. Labelling is a phenomenon familiarly used within the medical sphere, with the formulation of diagnoses and pathological classifications as an example. However, labelling can be hazardous, especially when the illness has the potential to be a focus for unwarranted stigma as in the case of mental illness.

Another aspect of interactionism is the analysis of institutionalisation. This is observed within hospital environments but also in other structures such as the armed forces, religious establishments and prisons. Life within an institution is bounded by the interactions between host and guest or doctor and patient. Institutions exist and succeed with adherence to rules, policy and regulation and insist upon compliance and docility from those within. Power and submission is crucial within an institution, and this dynamic may be observed within the doctor–patient relationship in hospitals where illness and seeking alleviation from symptoms depends upon the medical practitioner.

Perceptions of wellness and illness are central to the interactionist. There is a continuum of thought and behaviours extending from feeling unwell to seeking consultation. All of these stages are influenced by social factors and motivations as much as the symptoms of the disease. Seeking advice from health professionals is fraught with many variables that may prejudice the individual, some of which are attitudes of the health professional, age, gender, cost of treatment and employment pressure.

Marxist theory

Marxist theory can be explained as a capitalist social organisational belief. This model claims that illness and health are largely influenced by economic activity of the state, where power and inequality determines the ebb and flow of the workforce.

The core of Marxist conviction is that of conflict and struggle for the masses against the state, that there is no societal norm but a position of the dominant elite and subjugated underprivileged. This can be demonstrated by the work of Navarro (1986) who asserts health and medicine are supported and fed by capitalist structures determining the availability of treatment and accessibility of healthcare.

Marxists view many health problems as creations of the workplace, poverty and inequity; consequently stress and emotional problems are the construction of a capitalist drive for domination. Critics of this approach point out that Marxist health explanations fail to consider global and gender influences, and that it is too generalist and ignores individual experiences of illness.

Feminist theory

Feminist theory is embedded in the exposure of oppression and subjugation of women through the state, the roles women occupy and their financial oppression. This is achieved by controlling women's life opportunities and reproductivity, especially their disobedient bodies and minds. Feminist researchers voice the many differences in which health structures are gendered to the detriment of women. Historically this was ingrained in a belief that women's ailments were somehow traced to their reproductive inadequacies. Pregnancy and motherhood have been largely used as an example, revealing patriarchal medical interventions as seeking to control the nature and naturalness of birth. Where once women's bodies, sexuality and reproductive states were controlled by religion and dogma, today medicine has assumed authority.

The status of women and the burden of motherhood are given much breadth by contemporary feminist theorists, particularly Ann Oakley. She exposes the medical approach by highlighting how 'women's problems are constantly individualised: it is the individual woman who has the problem, and, even if many individual women have the same problem, the explanation of a defective psychology rather than a defective social structure is usually preferred' (Oakley 1993).

Gender is conceptualised as a powerful structural determinant of mental health, interacting with other variables including age, family structure, education, occupation, income and a variety of behavioural determinants of mental health. The emphasis on women's reproductive biology is likely to stem from the view that women's health is synonymous with and reducible to those illnesses or conditions related to their reproductive lifespan. However, Doyal (1995) believes in further complexity with the intertwining of domesticity, reproductivity and work outside of the home as determinants of women's health.

It has been identified that the level of psychological investment in relationships is pivotal in determining women's sense of self and self esteem (Jordan et al 1991). Theorists also argue that women generally subscribe to an ethic of care and consequently place a high degree of importance on the quality of their personal relationships. This investment places women at higher risk of disappointment and loss; if the woman requires reassurance and comfort without guarantee of fulfilment, she is at greater risk of emotional disappointment.

The way in which we mother our children is frequently examined within feminist research. Poverty, lack of opportunity for returning to work following childbirth, men occupying higher paid jobs, women undertaking the unpaid carer role for sick relatives and an overall sense of entrapment contributes to the subordination of women. Women are also exploited through the media. This has drawn criticism and condemnation from many feminist groups, and has been cited as responsible for increasing levels of body dysmorphia, eating disorders and quests for the 'body beautiful' (Jordanova 1995).

Stein (1997) describes women's health as inextricably bound in their social position. This is a factor that increases their vulnerability, sense of hopelessness and potential for mental illness. Women's position in society and their life opportunities (or lack of) forms the core of feminism; this dynamic creates tension and influences wellness and illness thus underpinning feminist belief systems.

Foucaldian theory

The final construct of social explanations of health and illness is the work of Michel Foucault, a French philosopher, social scientist and post-structuralist born in 1924. Foucault examines the concept of dominant medical discourse with constructed definitions of health and sickness, described as normality and deviance. This theory deconstructs elements of power and control specifically within medico-political structures.

Foucault was particularly interested in clinics and asylums, studying the way that discipline and control was crucial to the function and promotion of medicine. He also analysed the way that medicine manipulated and regulated people but also worked within the political systems ensuring its dominance.

Foucault examines the role of doctor and finds the purpose is to be objective, neutral and a classifier of symptoms, whereas the patient is viewed as a body with structures and systems waiting to give up answers. This objective surveillance of an organic composition is described as the 'clinical gaze' (Foucault 1973).

Foucault also identified the relationship of power and control between patient and health worker, and how medicine is a key player in controlling society and persuades the patient to acquiesce. The use of clinical examinations where the patient submits to physical assessment, where the findings are within the control of the assessor and may only be shared with the patient if the assessor chooses, describes the medical dominance. Furthermore, the classification of diseases is a construct that Foucault also exposes as part of the medical domination of society.

UNDERSTANDING THE CONCEPT OF SELF

The construction of wellness and illness may be explained through biomedical consideration. However, the mind is not an organ but a construct of experiences and emotions. To understand the mind is to determine who we are and how we came to be that person.

The development of self begins with the name our significant carers chose for us. Naming is not a neutral process, it is given with meaning and connects us to the family in which we are born. The development of self is dynamic and fluid, it consists of our perceptive self-awareness, the relationships we forge with others and feedback from those associations.

Perhaps deeper than this is the process of self-interaction, where we form reflexive and perceptive analysis of who we are and why we are. Mead (1934) identified this vibrant phenomenon and described language as a construct of this process, where the experience of self is nurtured by dialogue and interactions of those around us. The lives we lead and the way we present this information to the world through language forms the discourse of our life, and meaning and depth is reinforced by the level of reciprocity we gain from the world around us.

Labelling, stigma and a culture of blame

Mental illness may be described as losing part of one's 'self'.

Losing the sense of self is a powerful dynamic. It is easily taken especially if the individual is vulnerable and mentally ill. Losing one's identity may eventually be perceived as an irretrievable state for some, with the associated stigma seen as a response to a 'spoiled identity' (Goffman 1968). Having a label is to become that illness, to be known as a schizophrenic is to be stripped of individuality.

The experience of ill health and specifically the phenomenon of mental illness may be explained in terms of moral position. Society and science lay the blame for many diseases at the feet of those who are suffering. An example of this was seen when AIDS was declared, through sensationalistic media methods, as a punishment for living an immoral lifestyle. The medical profession uses lifestyle as an example of the burden upon health services and targets habits and behaviours as incurring disease and death, with smoking and obesity as exemplars. They also expose such practices as a public health concern leading to serious long-term health consequences with some treatments withheld on medico-moral grounds.

Using these analogies, it is relatively easy to understand concepts of blame and stigma surrounding mental illness. There is a societal belief that one can control emotions and the psyche. Therefore the descent into mental crisis is controllable and thus avoidable. When explaining to a doctor the symptoms of depression, it is common to describe feeling low, under the weather and a bit down. In reality, the symptoms are often acute and yet minimised to protect the listener. It is not surprising those suffering with mental health illnesses are often expected to 'pull themselves out of it' rather than have their feelings and experience taken seriously.

Some women experience mood lability during their reproductive cycle; the ebb and flow of hormonal changes induce emotional crises. This common occurrence is often under-reported and minimised by society but also the medical profession. Women describe being labelled as hormonal and suffering from PMT (premenstrual tension). For some, this emotional roller-coaster is more than a hormonal fluctuation, but rather a deluge of disturbing mood crises that the woman is plunged into with accepted regularity. The stigma and stereotyping associated with menstrual mood changes may prevent some women from accessing treatment and advice which could make their lives bearable.

Contemporary acceptance of postnatal depression is another example of how labelling a gendered illness provides society with a palatable disease brand and a range of treatment options. Traditionally, women were convinced their feelings were normal and they just had to get on with the emotional transition to motherhood. Those women who were psychotic were secretly separated from their families and infants, regularly institutionalised and subjected to barbaric treatments (Showalter 1987). Ironically, women were not only stigmatised by their illness but also by the removal of their child. The impact of this factor is immeasurable and in itself a contributory reason to slip further into a depressive fugue.

The concepts of stigma and stereotyping within mental illness are examined by Szasz (1994). Szasz (1962) was critical of the way psychiatry made assumptions about those labelled as mentally ill, arguing that in fact those individuals had problems in living and if their illness was a neurological abnormality then their illness should be organically attributable. Other anti-psychiatry theorists concur with Szasz (1994) and propose that many illnesses are in fact physical in which mental symptoms manifest. The experience of admission to psychiatric hospitals reinforces the labelling and stigma phenomenon. With the instigation of rules and an expectation of conformity from either self-regulation or medication, control is achieved.

To experience stigma is to be labelled as different. Scheff (1966) proposes that we develop ideas of mental illness, stigma and stereotyping when we are very young, and that these concepts are reinforced by the power of the media. Fear is a powerful instrument feeding society's aversion to those who are different. If children are exposed to images of monsters and mad men, their inherent beliefs as adults will guide their judgements. However, if stigma is understood as a reaction to difference then the process is more an assimilation of society's rules and regulations adopted by medicine and the state. There is even some mileage in the notion that mental health symptoms are just another form of identity markers like sexuality, ethnicity, class and age. Who does not hear the voice of reason and see those they have just lost to death? Many people see and hear strange things and yet are not diagnosed schizophrenic.

The effects of power and control cannot be underestimated in the lives of vulnerable people; there is no greater susceptibility than mental illness within this dynamic. These theoretical methodologies, explored from a sociological perspective, challenge the dominance of medical discourse and the use of power and knowledge to which it subscribes.

PSYCHOLOGICAL APPROACHES TO UNDERSTANDING MENTAL ILLNESS

Understanding mental health within a psychological domain is fraught with difficulties. There are many facets to this area that conflict with others. Feminists would argue it is impossible to view women's mental well-being through one singular model because of the historical context of some of the theorists, for example Freud (1926).

The forerunner of modern psychological theorists is Wilhelm Wundt (Psi Cafe 1999). He investigated the mind in an approach described as introspection, which sought to analyse and reach understanding of the structure of consciousness, calling this model structuralism. However, it could be argued that it is impossible to actually get inside the mind and be reassured of the accuracy of scientific findings. Therefore, the consensus must be that introspection is largely subjective and individual-specific.

It is worthwhile looking at the major influences of psychology, psychoanalysis and psychotherapy that may in turn give depth and insight to some contemporary mental health issues. There are many theoretical perspectives that seek to explain human development and robust arguments to support all. For the purpose of this work, four domains will be explored:

1. The behaviourist approach
2. The psychodynamic approach
3. The cognitive approach
4. The humanist approach.

All of these approaches are seminal in seeking to understand and explain the secrets of human development and functioning and it is important to understand how each influences current thinking within mental illness.

The behaviourist approach

This model may be explained as the mechanistic representation of two interrelated theories – behaviourism and social learning theory. The behaviourist model describes mental disorder as an internal dysfunction due to an underlying physical cause. Areas explored by behaviourists include imagery and memory association, language, moral and gender development and free will.

By researching people and behaviour in environmentally controlled situations, those who subscribe to behavioural theory see human development as quantitative and continuous. This perspective focuses upon the impact of experience and how it affects behaviour by deconstructing complex stimuli. Those behavioural responses are examined, measured and recorded with no interest in interpretive value; the basis is scientific quantitative evidence. This theory forms the foundations of the current medical model that uses randomised controlled situations to prove treatment efficacy.

The behaviourist perspective is best known by the work and views of Pavlov (1927) who described the term 'conditioning'. Conditioning is separated into two domains: operant and classical. Classical conditioning is a type of learning, responding to a stimulus not necessarily associated with the experience. Pavlov famously experimented with dog's salivation responses to demonstrate how classical conditioning worked. This theory forms the basis for the cognitive behavioural approach to contemporary therapy, often used in conditions such as obsessive compulsive disorder and phobias.

Skinner (1938) moved the theory from classical conditioning to that of operant conditioning. He proposed that human behaviour can be predicted and controlled, although he deduced this from his work with non-humans. However, his theory did not allow for what individuals think, which in turn may determine what they do. Skinner maintained that behaviour is controlled by three consequences: 'positive' and 'negative reinforcers', which generally support behaviour, and 'punishers', which lead to avoidance. This theory translates well into human behaviour patterns where an individual might experience a traumatic event and exhibit stress and anxiety or withdraw to cope with life.

Case study: SONIA

Sonia has had a particularly traumatic birth but is unable to express her distressing experience and does not mentally process the event. She suffers from nightmares and hypervigilance. She manages to continue with life and blocks out the experience until 1 day about 6 months later, she finds herself on the top deck of a bus which is diverted from its normal route and takes her past the hospital where she gave birth. On seeing the signs for the hospital, she experiences panic, somatic sensations and begins to vomit. Sonia's response was triggered by the unexpected sight of the hospital (stimuli stressors) where she had given birth. Fear signals were activated and she reacted physically to unprocessed trauma. This can be explained as classical conditioning.

The behaviourist approach is a persuasive perspective on human behaviour, but while convincing in terms of measurable events and scientific psychology, it fails to interpret meaningful interaction. Frequency of behaviour does not in itself tell us a great deal about why we do things. Language and communication are greater mechanisms by which to appreciate the significance of experience. Despite criticism, this model has become influential and is frequently used to address maladaptive behaviours through techniques such as cognitive behavioural therapy.

The psychodynamic approach

The psychodynamic theory of mental illness might be explained as a dysfunction of internal factors caused by deep psychological conflict. This model may be interpreted using a deterministic stance whereby human nature and personality are explained as driven by instinct and impulses.

It is probable that one of the greatest original thinkers of how the personality determines our behaviour is Sigmund Freud. Freud (1926) developed the theory of unconscious conflict, which he described as unconscious thoughts that struggle and emerge within the deepest structures of human personality. He also brought to our attention the concept of hysteria and proposed its roots were bound in unresolved unconscious conflicts that begin in childhood.

Freud is closely connected with psychodynamic theory and the practice of psychoanalysis. The context of this perspective is that most of what we are conscious of is just a small part of what we have hidden. Freud called these concepts the 'pre-conscious' thoughts not accessible at that moment and the 'unconscious' or thoughts that are wholly inaccessible. Freud proposed that much of what is unconscious is repressed memory, experiences which were so unpleasant that the mind puts them out of reach of conscious awareness. These unconscious thoughts can be made available though techniques such as free association, dream interpretation, hypnosis and transference. The practice by which the unconscious is raised and explored in the conscious mind is known as psychoanalysis.

Within the psychodynamic perspective, the personality is thought to be composed of three cooperate structures (Freud 1923/1984):

1. The id: present at birth, is impulsive and pleasure seeking
2. The ego: helps to cope with the world, deals with reality
3. The superego: concerned with moral judgements and feelings.

Freud also believed that all mental dysfunction may be explained through this framework and that individuals construct defence mechanisms as a way of dealing with anxiety and stress. Defence mechanisms in turn prevent repressed thoughts from entering our consciousness and protect the individual, but distorting their reality.

The work of Freud and other psychoanalysts has received great interest and much criticism. Disparagement is levelled at Freud's research, which was restricted to young women and lacked scientific rigour. Despite this, Freud remains a significant marker in our understanding of personality and internal psychological human functioning.

The cognitive approach

While very much in alignment with the behaviourist model, cognitive theory is fixed in the notion that certain behaviours can be adapted by observing them – social learning theory.

Bandura (1971) describes this concept as observational learning. This methodology draws closely on links between behavioural and cognitive dysfunction. There is still a strong connection between internal processes but it is primordially focussed upon thoughts, expectations and attitudes contributing to mental disorder.

Beck (1967) describes some of these dysfunctional thought processes as cognitive errors and attributes mental disorder as a product of faulty thinking. Therefore, individuals must be able to rectify and change behaviour. Beck understands depression through this model, explaining that most depressed people see the world in a negative way and view themselves in a pessimistic self-fulfilling manner. This description of illogical thinking includes:

- Magnification and minimisation – amplifying difficulties while playing down achievements
- Selective abstraction – selecting one factor rather than others
- Arbitrary inference – arriving at a decision without any supporting evidence
- Over generalisation – sweeping statement using trivial facts.

While this approach is convincing, there is criticism from behaviourists for its lack of scientific rigour and unempirical position, whereas humanists argue that humanity is more complex than can be explained as just thoughts and processes.

The humanist approach

Humanism emerged in strength and popularity as a response to the reductionist behavioural approach. One leading intellectual in this theoretical field is Abraham Maslow (1968). He introduced a 'Hierarchy of Needs' and the concept of self-actualisation as the highest level of human attainment in a desire for personal growth. The principle of Maslow's hierarchy is based upon a variety of requirements that need to be met for our satisfaction. These are separated into physiological, psychological and finally self-actualisation, which is the realisation of our true potential. Critics of Maslow's ideas state it is impossible to define self-actualisation, since it is uniquely individual and therefore impossible to test or measure. However, at the heart of Maslow's theory was the belief that free will is a distinct characteristic of humanity, with the ability to choose and therefore how to respond.

The humanistic model interprets the world using a phenomenological framework. This is subjective and individual specific in contrast to a behaviourist interpretation (which is rooted in objectivity and focuses upon dysfunctional behaviours). Humanistic principles assume people are inherently good and strive for personal growth, dignity and self-determination. This model also proposes that mental health cannot be defined as the absence of symptoms or explained as the adjustment to societal norms but as the full realisation of our true potential. This may mean to be fully at one with humankind and the world in which we exist – to be creative, and to experience life as it is without egotistic pursuit. Mental illness thus arises because external factors block personal growth and potential.

Rogers (1951) researched meticulously the 'person centred' therapy approach, which has contributed immensely to the modern therapy world. Rogers identified the issue of self-concept, and the impact of the therapeutic connection as measurable and influential within the therapy relationship. In the person-centred approach to therapy, it is the values of the client that are held as the core to healing. This model is non-directive and structured around rephrasing a client's responses and looks to the client for their feelings in the 'here and now'. Rogers (1980) also states there are three core elements to encourage personal growth in therapy – genuineness, unconditional positive regard and empathy. These core conditions are applied as techniques in the therapy relationship. Empathic understanding is achieved by active listening that seeks not only to hear clearly what clients bring, but also in understanding the feelings behind the words. Rogers argues that the client has vast internal resources to facilitate personal change if given the necessary environment, the attitude of the therapist and expansion of self-understanding.

CONTEMPORARY APPROACHES AND TREATMENTS TO MENTAL ILLNESS

In the past, those experiencing mental illness have received bizarre and often inhuman treatment approaches, without benefit to society and the individual. Modern treatment has the benefit of a pharmaceutical explosion and a shift into humanistic talking therapies. Current service provision and treatment approaches to mental health are based upon the concept of symptom classification. This method forms the foundation of the DSM-IV (American Psychiatric Association 1991), although neither the DSM-IV nor the ICD 10 (WHO 1994) uses mental illness as a descriptor but instead adopts the term mental disorder (Table 2.1).

The DSM-IV recommends using Axes I, II and III consistently, but Axes IV and V are optional. This method of classification, diagnosis and labelling is difficult because mental illness is often described subjectively and symptoms experienced uniquely. This method of classification is also criticised for its assumptions about human and social functioning, family life and ethnocentricity.

Public health approach to mental well–being

Mental health is described as 'a state of complete physical, mental and social well-being and not merely the absence of disease or infirmity' (WHO 1981). However, it is evident that improving mental health is a key priority for all societies and requires approaches that acknowledge this concept. Redressing the balance between physical and mental well-being is the core of modern public health strategies, particularly since it has been established that many physical illnesses are either caused or complicated by dysfunctional mental health.

Public health is based upon social and political strategies that expose social determinants of health and illness by redressing inequalities using education and health promotion. Adopting a public health model to address mental health is persuasive, since it acknowledges the complexity of its illness aetiology. Health promotion is one means by which public health is achieved, putting the onus upon the individual but also reaching a wider population. There is a collaborative approach across many sectors including economic, health, education, environmental and social care. Applying this thinking to mental health challenges classification and diagnostic models, as it clearly recognises that mental well-being is a dynamic process and a continuum.

This notion fits with meaningfulness and a sense of gaining control over life, or sense of coherence as defined by Antonovsky (1987). However, while a public health approach draws upon the public's willingness and engagement, there still exists a need for treatment in some cases that self-motivation cannot fulfil.

Pharmacological treatments

Drug treatments for mental illness largely fall into four categories:

1. Anxiolytics
2. Antidepressants
3. Antipsychotics
4. Mood stabilisers.

Anxiolytics are more commonly known as anti-anxiety drugs. This group of drugs includes minor tranquillisers used to treat anxiety states, although they may also be used for inducing sleep. Anxiolytics are efficacious when used briefly but may cause problems when used for longer periods of time. This group of drugs are known to be addictive, hence they are prescribed for short periods only. Discontinuation may also induce the symptoms they are designed to reduce, described as the rebound effect.

Antidepressants are prescribed for persistent low mood and other symptoms of depression. While these drugs are not addictive, they are associated with a range of side-effects. First generation antidepressants are monoamine oxidase inhibitors (MAOIs) and tricyclics. However, MAOIs are rarely used today because of substance interactions, for example with meat and dairy products. Side-effects of tricyclics are wide ranging and this group of antidepressants are predominantly toxic in overdose. New generation antidepressants are selective serotonin reuptake inhibitors (SSRIs) and serotonin and noradrenaline (norepinephrine) reuptake inhibitors (SNRIs). This new group of antidepressants are less sedating and potentially less toxic than tricyclics. They can cause nausea, diarrhoea and vomiting and more occasionally other adverse effects such as headaches, restlessness, anxiety and disturbed sexual function. These drugs may be useful for treating eating disorders and some obsessive–compulsive conditions, as well as depression.

Tolerance to antidepressants increases with the progression of treatment, generally starting with a low dose and increasing as symptoms allow. It is normal to remain on antidepressant therapy for at least 6 months, even with mood improvement to avoid relapse. Stopping treatment is usually gradual and under the guidance of health professionals.

Antipsychotic drugs known as neuroleptics are used to treat schizophrenia, manic phase of bipolar disorder and other psychotic conditions. These drugs are not tranquillisers and not addictive.

They may help to reduce agitation but often cause drowsiness. Antipsychotics are useful in relieving auditory hallucinations, as well as delusions, such as paranoia. Long-term use of these drugs frequently causes distressing side-effects, including movement disorders or extrapyramidal symptoms. These long-term effects may make taking medication orally difficult, however depot injections are used to overcome this.

Atypical antipsychotics work differently and cause fewer side-effects. Atypical antipsychotics include risperidone and clozapine and are classed as new generation drugs. Clozapine can cause a reduction in white blood cell production and therefore regular blood screening is recommended. Risperidone may also be used as an injection where there is difficulty in taking oral medication.

Mood-stabilisers can be used to treat bipolar affective disorder and severe depression. Lithium is commonly used and extremely effective in the treatment of severe bipolar affective disorder. However, overdose can be toxic at low levels, therefore blood screening is carried out on a regular basis. The side-effects of this group of drugs are few and therapeutic response usually good. However, lithium is known to cause congenital abnormalities of the fetal heart and therefore a careful risk benefit analysis should be undertaken if this drug is used during the early stages of pregnancy.

Electroconvulsive therapy (ECT) may also be used where depressive symptoms are enduring and unresponsive to pharmacological management. ECT generates a degree of fear and mystery in the public domain, however treatment is considered effective in many cases and may be used for treating serious depression.

Talking therapies

While pharmacological treatments are widely used and commonly known in the public domain, there is increasing acknowledgement that talking and gaining personal insight motivates change in those with a broad range of mental health problems.

There has been an explosion in counselling and psychotherapeutic interventions in this decade with therapy widely available to all and not just the wealthy. In the last few decades, Americans developed a love affair with their therapists and though the reserved British character may be more inhibited when sharing feelings, there is no doubt that talking is gaining strength as a treatment.

With this shift from medical approaches in resolving mental crisis, many health workers are encouraged to develop skills in counselling techniques, especially cognitive behavioural and brief therapy models. NICE (2003) evaluated this model of treatment as favourable in mild to moderately depressed patients and recommend that psychotherapeutic support outweighs pharmacological benefit.

Counselling and psychotherapy is undergoing regulation ensuring quality and rigour to the patient and professional experience. There are many models of talking therapies, e.g. cognitive behavioural, person centred, integrative, Gestalt, etc. However, they are best matched by the problem the client brings to the potential and philosophical beliefs of the therapist. It may be confusing that counselling and psychotherapy are described dually, however it is generally accepted that:

- Counselling refers to enabling free and expressive discussion about distress in the 'here and now' without therapist intervention, fitting with Rogers' model of person-centred counselling (1951)
- Psychotherapy is the dynamic interpretation of thoughts, dreams and feelings that are buried. The level of current distress is considered to be part of a deeper suppressed experience that has emerged in a current situation. This therapy is psychodynamic and is embedded in Freud's work (1984).

There are also many new techniques emerging from integration of models, e.g. eye movement desensitisation and reprocessing (EMDR); neuro-linguistic programming (NLP); hypnotherapy; systemic therapy – the list is long and is growing. This expansion is a response to public demand and a search for an alternative to pharmacology.

Holistic therapies

Holism and holistic therapies have stood the test of time and continue into the twenty-first century with vitality and interest. Holism incorporates the normative to the extraordinary in embracing 'if it works then it is acceptable'. Some commonly known holistic therapies are:

- Aromatherapy
- Massage
- Reflexology

- Homeopathy
- Neurofeedback
- Art, music, dance therapy
- Nutritional therapy.

The message is that one size does not fit all. Holism seeks to embrace the dynamic aspects of the human condition by balancing emotional, mental, spiritual and physical elements of each person, concentrating on the cause of the illness as well as symptoms.

CONCLUSION

Mental well-being and disorder are arbitrary states. Although it may be impossible to be sure about the definitions and origins of mental illness, one thing is certain – we will all experience some aspect of mental dysfunction. Global statistics hold this problem high on the international agenda and highlight the burden it places on health services. The economic cost of mental illness is inestimable, and therefore understanding the issues and hearing the realities is crucial to moving forward.

There are many theories and convincing arguments for why mental health is an issue and how understanding the aetiology may help to redress the problems. Nevertheless, theory often fails reality. Controlling the problem by social and structural means is contentious and has failed in the past with arguable moral consequences.

The impact of living with mental illness is felt far wider than with the individual; it resonates in families, localities and society in general. There are consequences to mental illness such as stigma, stereotyping and labelling often reducing life opportunities for the individual. More women than men are at risk of some form of mental illness in their lifetime and so gender-sensitive treatments and services are essential. Childbirth is a window of opportunity for both women and health professionals. This time should be seized upon to ensure previous mental health issues are acknowledged and treatment is offered in ways that are acceptable to women, but also that any distress during this time is treated with the respect and dignity it deserves.

References

American Psychiatric Association 1991 Diagnostic and statistical manual of mental disorders, 4th edn. American Psychiatric Association, Washington

Antonovsky A 1987 Unraveling the mystery of health. Jossey-Bass, San Francisco

Bandura A 1971 Social learning theory. General Learning Press, New Jersey

Beck A 1967 Depression: causes and treatments. University of Philadelphia Press, Philadelphia

Blumer H 1969 Symbolic interactionism: perspective and method. Prentice-Hall, New Jersey

Doyal L 1995 What makes women sick: gender and the political economy of health. Macmillan, London

Goffman E 1968 Stigma: notes on the management of spoiled identity. Penguin, Harmondsworth

Foucault M 1973 The birth of the clinic. Tavistock, London

Freud S 1923/1984 The ego and the id. Pelican Freud Library (11), Harmondsworth

Freud S 1926 Inhibition, symptoms and anxiety. Standard edition of the complete psychological works of Sigmund Freud, Vol 20. Hogarth Press, London

Jordan J, Kaylan A, Surrey J L 1991 Women's growth in connection: writings from the Stone Centre. Guilford Publications, New York

Jordanova, L J 1995 The social construction of medical knowledge. Social History of Medicine 8:361–381

Laing R D 1967 The politics of experience and the bird of paradise. Penguin, London

Maslow A 1968 Towards a psychology of being, 2nd edn. Harper & Row, New York

Mead G H 1934 Mind, self and society. Morris C W (ed.) University of Chicago Press, Chicago

Mora G 1980 Historical and theoretical trends in psychiatry. In: Kaplan HI, Freedman AM, Sadock BJ (eds) Comprehensive textbook of psychiatry III. Williams & Wilkins, Baltimore

Navarro, V 1986 Crisis, health, and medicine: a social critique. Tavistock, London

National Institute for Clinical Excellence 2003 Clinical guideline depression: the management of depression in primary and secondary care. NICE, London

Nishizawa S, Benkelfat C, Young S N, et al. 1997 Differences between males and females in rates of serotonin synthesis in human brain. Proceedings of the National Academy of Sciences of the United States of America 94(10):4823–4824

Oakley A 1993 Essays on women, medicine and health. Edinburgh University Press, Edinburgh

Parsons T 1951 The social system. Free Press, New York

Pavlov I P 1927 Conditioned reflexes. Oxford University Press, London

Psi Cafe 1999 Wundt Wilhem. Online. Available: http://www.psy.pdx.edu/PsiCafe/KeyTheorists/Wundt.htm

Rogers C R 1951 Client-centred therapy: its current practice, implications and theory. Houghton-Mifflin, Boston

Rogers C R 1980 A way of being. Houghton-Mifflin, Boston

Scheff T 1966 Being mentally ill: a sociological theory. Aldine, Chicago

Showalter E 1987 The female malady: women, madness and English culture, 1830–1980. Virago Press, London

Skinner B F 1938 The behaviour of organisms. Appleton-Century-Crofts, New York

Stein J 1997 Empowerment and women's health: theory, methods and practice. Zed Books, London

Szasz T S 1962 The myth of mental illness. Harper & Row, New York

Szasz T S 1994 Cruel compassion – psychiatric control of society's untreated. Wiley, New York

University of Virginia Health System 1998 Twenty medical classics of the Jefferson era. William Cullen (1710–1790) First lines of the practice of physic. Online. Available: http://www.med.virginia.edu/hs-library/historical/classics/Cullen.html

Waitzkin H 1971 Latent functions of the sick role in various institutional settings. Social Science and Medicine 5:45–75

World Health Organization 1981 Social dimensions of mental health (5). WHO, Geneva

World Health Organization 1994 International classification of disease (10). WHO, Geneva

Chapter 3

Promoting mental well-being
Jennifer Hall

INTRODUCTION

The aim of this chapter is to explore the concept of women's mental health from the angle of the whole person and her needs and apply this to pregnancy and childbirth. Since its inception, the National Health Service (NHS) in the UK has had an approach that has divided people into individual conditions or diseases. Departments in NHS trusts are labelled according to the parts of the body that are not functioning and medical practitioners and, to an extent, nurses choose to specialise in particular areas according to these labels. The difficulty in this approach lies in addressing the individual's needs according to their separate parts. For the professionals concerned their focus will also be upon the specialisms in which they are functioning. This approach may mean a system is treated without dealing with an alternative or underlying cause for the problem. Peters (2005) suggests that a medical model approach to mental health can disempower individuals while prompting society to ignore the personal and social aspects of mental distress. Instead a holistic approach to mental health aims to meet all the needs of the person and bring complete healing.

HEALTH AND WELL-BEING

The concept of health is an individual one. To each person, their idea of being 'healthy' will be dependent on a number of things including the concepts they learnt within families while growing up and the social and cultural group to which they belong. The World Health Organization's definition of health states that it 'is a state of complete physical, mental and social well-being and not

merely the absence of disease or infirmity' (WHO 1948). This definition demonstrates the need to have a holistic understanding of
people's needs in order to provide the most appropriate care and
to promote health. Holistic care involves caring for the individual
as a whole person and recognising the interlinking of the elements
of body, mind and spirit that make up the person. It is also taking
into consideration the social world in which that person is placed,
which includes the impact of generational and cultural influences.

There is evidence to show that social deprivation has an effect on
both the physical (Poulton et al 2002) and emotional state of a
person (Skapinakis et al 2005). There is also evidence to suggest
that a physically ill person may have mental health issues or that
someone with a mental disorder may manifest physical symptoms.
In addition, understanding how the spirit of the person pervades
every facet of their being (Swinton 2001:16) will lead to a realisation of how a mental or physical illness may lead to a spiritual need
as well (Dombeck 1996), or how spiritual distress may manifest
within the other areas.

WOMEN'S HEALTH

Globally, women's health is seen as a particular issue of need (WHO
2000). It is suggested that a major depressive disorder is experienced by around 7–13% of women worldwide (Bennett et al 2004).
The factors of inequality, poverty, violence and overwork play an
important role in creating challenge with women's health (WHO
2000). In particular, women's mental health is viewed as a specific
need affected by the above social issues, but also by biological
factors related to gender (Burt & Hendrick 1997:3). In taking a holistic approach to separate the issues of mental health from the rest of
a woman's persona or social life would be inappropriate. It is therefore necessary to provide a focus on mental health that will value
the whole person, as indicated by Peters (2005). Approaching care
in this way will mean that women's health needs will be met appropriately. If the cause of mental health difficulties are related to social
need, steps can be taken to reduce this. Further if the underlying
cause is physical, as in relation to thyroid disease (Timms 2003),
the condition may be treated effectively. Purely treating the
mental health issue with medicine may also be inappropriate and
the use of complementary therapies (Bastard & Tiran 2006), alternative therapies such as exercise (Hawkins 2005a), light therapies

(Hawkins 2005b), herbs (Hawkins 2005b) or prayer or meditation (Koenig 2005:97–98) may bring results.

HEALTH PROMOTION IN RELATION TO MENTAL HEALTH

The World Health Organization's understanding of health, as quoted above, notes that good health is not just related to the absence of illness but a sense of wholeness, and an interaction between the different components of a person. Mental well-being therefore is wholeness of the mental state of the person. The Health Education Authority (1997) has defined it in terms of:

- Emotional and spiritual resilience giving the ability to enjoy life and to cope with pain, disappointment and sadness
- A positive sense of well-being and an underlying belief in our own, and other's dignity and worth.

Swinton (2001:35) suggests there are seven elements that define mental health:

1. Absence of illness
2. Appropriate social behaviour
3. Freedom from worry and guilt
4. Personal competence and control
5. Self-acceptance and self-actualisation
6. Unification and organisation of personality
7. Open-mindedness and flexibility.

These definitions illustrate the focus on the individual. However, in the political arena, the health of the individual is applied in a wider setting. The European Union (EU) states that an individual's mental health 'enables them to realise their intellectual and emotional potential and to find and fulfil their roles in social, school and working life' (Commission of the European Communities, CEC 2005:4). Any form of promotion of good mental health will involve aiming to enable a person to achieve the above goals. Mental health promotion is high on the current political agenda in the UK. The National Service Framework for mental health (Department of Health, DoH 1999) states that 'mental health promotion involves any action to enhance the mental well-being of individuals, families, organisations and communities'. Standard 1 of the framework aims to 'ensure that health and social services promote mental health and reduce the discrimination and social exclusion associated with mental health problems'. To achieve this, health and social services are expected to:

- Promote mental health for all, working with individuals and communities
- Combat discrimination against individuals and groups with mental health problems and promote their social inclusion.

This means that any strategies that aim to improve mental well-being should have a wider remit than just the individual and should involve a multidisciplinary approach. Promoting value of all persons within society will mean that those who are currently marginalised socially, which leads to symptoms of low-esteem, and then ultimately to mental ill health, should feel included, supported and subsequently empowered. Currently, the professional boundaries between medical doctors, psychiatrists, nurses and those who work with alternative or complementary approaches to health create different tiers of systems and fragmented support. The progress toward interdisciplinary learning, where the boundaries of the roles become more blurred increases knowledge of responsibilities and is suggested will also enable greater understanding and better future working in practice (Pullon & Fry 2005). However, Robinson & Cottrell (2005) have demonstrated that there remain issues of identity among professionals in establishing team working. Psychiatrists are particularly powerful within the organisation of the maternity services (Brimblecombe 2004). Breaking down barriers to create multidisciplinary teams with effective communication will have added value for communities whose need is greatest.

The current fragmented nature of mental healthcare has been starkly illustrated by the CEMACH report (National Institute for Clinical Excellence, NICE et al 2004). The issue of lack of communication between medical doctors, psychiatrists and midwives has led to women not being supported and treated effectively in times of mental crisis.

Case study

'A professional woman died from violent means, together with baby and another child. At the booking clinic she revealed a family history of mental illness but denied any personal psychiatric history. Her GP records contained the evidence that she had taken several previous overdoses and had been treated previously by a psychiatrist but this was not shared with her maternity care providers. There were no concerns about her mental health until the very end of pregnancy when she called her GP saying that she was unable to leave the house. She was diagnosed with agoraphobia and was referred to the community mental health team. She declined psychological intervention on the unusual grounds that the resultant anxiety would harm the baby. This was accepted and no arrangements were made for her to be seen again. Following her death, the family revealed that the woman had wished them to conceal her previous history and that she was developing a paranoid psychosis'.

NICE et al (2004:168)

It was stated in the report that note should have been taken of her previous psychiatric and family histories and referral made to the appropriate agencies. Further if this information had been passed on to the other community carers, recognition of the agoraphobia late in pregnancy as a serious factor may have enabled more prompt action.

The EU also includes the mental well-being of the individual in society enables contribution 'to prosperity, solidarity and social justice' (CEC 2005:4). The financial implications of improving the mental well-being of the individual is also highlighted by ensuring incorporation of mental healthcare with general healthcare and reducing the length of time as hospital in-patients (CEC 2005:4). It is recognised that the effectiveness of mental health promotion is increased through combined strategies that deal both with the individual needs and community issues that may weaken mental health (DoH 1999:15). A benefit of having this approach will mean that the mental health needs of all in the community may be met, rather than just the individual who is known as having a particular need. There will also be an impact on those who have not been identified as having mental health needs. Encouraging a greater value on mental well-being will have a long-term effect with the potential improvement in physical well-being (Goodwin et al 2000). There should be recognition that a particular construction of society may have a potentially positive effect on mental well-being. Koenig's (2005) recent review of studies relating to religious communities and mental illness demonstrates that the majority showed there is a benefit in having a religious belief. It appears that the support that people receive from being within a community, as well as wanting to help others, and having a sense of gratitude, are factors of the benefit of having a faith.

The use of artistic expression as an outlet for mental health is reported as valuable (Morris 2002). It is also known that the improvement of physical working environments through better design and use of art may have a positive effect on the well-being of both patients and staff (Waller & Finn 2004). Furthermore, the style of physical environmental living conditions may have a profound effect on mental health (Galea et al 2005). These projects could be transferred into communities where the environment could be transformed to enhance the well-being of all who live and work there. The issues may be explored further in maternity services to ensure the environments for care may ultimately be improved (Newburn 2006).

Policy review of the National Health Service demonstrated that the public have asked for more recognition and care for emotional and mental health (DoH 2006). This has led to a vision for mental well-being that sees this being carried out at community level (Sainsbury Centre for Mental Health 2006). With maternity services based primarily in the community, the role of the midwife in mental health promotion will be increased.

HEALTH PROMOTION AND MIDWIVES

In recent years midwives have been exploring the concept of salutogenesis (Antonovsky 1993) as a way of understanding and examining health. This method of promoting health is viewed as a holistic method, where people are 'negotiators' of the process (Royal College of Midwives, RCM 2002). It involves establishing their ability to recognise that life has meaning, the resources they have to manage the demands of life and the degree to which a person comprehends the meanings, order and consistency of their life (RCM 2002). The place of the person in society, culture, their family and community is seen as important. This clearly lies within the political agenda.

The role of promoting the well-being of clients has become a greater responsibility for health carers. Government policy in the UK to create a health service that acts with an increased preventative focus has recently been introduced (DoH 2005). This aims to reduce poverty and unemployment rates as well as improve environmental conditions. The key aims of health professionals will include:

- Better management of blood pressure and cholesterol levels by GPs
- Implementation of National Institute for Health and Clinical Excellence guidance on cancer treatment
- Reducing smoking during pregnancy and adult smoking prevalence as a whole
- Increasing the uptake of breastfeeding
- Tackling childhood obesity
- Reducing under 18 pregnancy and improving access to sexual health services
- Improving mental health and well-being and reducing suicide rates.

Areas within this list clearly fall into the remit of the midwife. However, the public health role is thought to have a wider perspective. Before the advent of this policy, midwives have been involved in promotion of health. The role has been viewed as (RCM 2001):

- Encompassing the roots and causes of health and ill health, as well as its treatment
- Seeing health within its overall social and political context, rather than as an isolated medical event
- Looking for solutions in wider social action, individual empowerment and community development, as well as in clinical interventions.

Further, Kaufmann (2002) gives pointers of:

- Making women empowered
- Promotion of midwifery philosophy of care
- Working for health, not just providing healthcare
- Developing wider alliances and working in partnerships
- Tackling health inequalities.

This illustrates that the midwife has an important place in promoting the well-being of women. Where women may often be marginalised in societies, midwives will have a place in acting as support and advocate and meeting social needs as well as the physical and emotional. There should be recognition of the interplay between these elements and the need for a holistic approach.

Empowerment and mental well-being

The unique relationship of the woman and midwife has the potential role of enabling women to achieve positive mental well-being. Strategies in place may lead to psychological resilience and greater ability to cope. Poor mental health has been linked to poor self-esteem and deficient self-worth (WHO 2001:11). The lack of self-esteem may be the cause of mental health problems or it may occur the other way round. Enabling a person to be empowered and to increase self-esteem will promote mental well-being. This has been recognised in schemes to provide advocacy and support to promote empowerment (WHO 2004). This links to the role of the midwife who has a place as acting as advocate for childbearing women. The role also includes empowering women in making choices and promoting self esteem and self worth. Effectiveness of the midwife in this role will promote mental well-being for the woman. Conversely, the midwife acting in a way that is less than empowering may also negatively affect a person's mental health significantly. A study in Iceland demonstrated how midwives perceived as 'caring' were viewed as empowering for the women whereas those who were thought of as uncaring were seen as discouraging (Halldorsdottir & Karlsdottir 1996). Powell Kennedy (2000) further demonstrated that women perceived that the midwives had a specific role of enabling them to achieve their goals.

Other ways women may be empowered are through advocacy or working with groups of similar women. Maternity services groups, such as the National Childbirth Trust and Association for the Improvement of the Maternity Service, have historically enabled and empowered women to make appropriate choices. These groups have grown up through the lack of trust women have had of the organisation and structure of the maternity services, including midwifery practice. For some midwives, working outside the structure of the NHS as independent midwives enables them to work autonomously according to the rules of practice and to truly act as advocates for women.

Promoting a philosophy of women-centred care

The philosophy of women-centred care has been promoted since the advent of the 'Changing Childbirth' report (DoH 1993). Ten years on, the National Services Framework echoed the principles of the report and indicated a need for change in the maternity services to aim to meet the needs of the individual women (DoH 2004). Current reduced levels of maternity service staff is making the ideals laid down in the framework a difficulty. However, midwives have a responsibility to examine personal practices and to address areas where care may be improved.

Historically the organisation and structures of the maternity service have led to women being disempowered. The move away from community-based services into centralised units in the 1970s and 1980s led to women feeling they were on a 'production line' and increased the amount of technology being utilised. The effect of the lack of individual care and support and the perceived lack of value for women may have had a significant effect on mental health issues. Increased anxiety levels and stress, fear and lack of control may be perpetuated by bringing women out of communities with which they are familiar into large clinical hospital units where they rarely see the same caregiver. The 'Know-your-midwife' scheme (Flint & Poulangeris 1986) in the 1980s demonstrated that care could be constructed differently. A group of women were cared for during pregnancy, birth and postnatally by a team of four midwives. Consequently, they saw fewer caregivers and appeared to be more emotionally satisfied with the experience. Since that study, some areas have introduced team care with mixed success. In some cases, construction of the teams was too large to enable the continuity described by Flint, or management gave too large a case load for the group care to be effective. In other areas, one-to-one schemes have been introduced, with midwives working in pairs, demonstrating satisfaction for both women and their carers (McCourt et al 1998). The development of birth centres that provide a home-from-home atmosphere have been created in recognition of the psychological effect of bringing women into cold, clinical maternity units and as a social model of care (Kirkham 2003). The principle is that increasing satisfaction with maternity care will promote well-being in the woman and her family.

Working for health

The importance of the health promotion role should be recognised by midwives. Though there is currently limited working towards health pre-conceptually, midwives can discover important issues in pregnancy or beyond, that may have an effect on future pregnancies.

Partnership working

Midwives have been notorious in trying to stand their ground with regard to their professional roles. The concept of women-centred care has been addressed already and there is still a need for recognition of the woman and her family as partners in care. In the case of mental health issues, self-knowledge of the woman of previous experience, as well as that of her close family should be taken into consideration when planning appropriate support for care. Inclusiveness will promote mental well-being through recognition of respect and autonomy for the individual and ensuring power remains with the person concerned.

Midwives are also part of a multidisciplinary workforce. There is a need to ensure communication between the professions is effective, especially in relation to mental health issues, as raised through the CEMACH report (NICE 2004). Valuing the roles of the other professions through understanding and team-working is vital. At the same time, there is a need to value groups that have a specific role in supporting women. Recognising the availability of local resources will enable appropriate community support to be utilised at the time when it is most needed. Women may also choose to use alternative or complementary therapies and the midwife working in partnership with these practitioners can enable a holistic approach to the women's needs.

Tackling health inequalities

Throughout the world, community-based midwives are often intimately aware of the situations in which women live. As guests in a woman's home, they are able to witness her living conditions, her belongings, her other family members and the area in which she lives. This role means that the midwife is in a position to recognise extreme hardship or squalor that may have an impact on the health and well-being of the mother and the unborn infant. Those who have mental health problems are often living in the worst conditions. To this end, midwives then have a responsibility to act as advocate for the woman and her family with other agencies who may be in a position to offer greater support. Team working with community leaders, councils or social services may mean that greater support is available for the whole community, not just the individual pregnant woman. Projects such as 'Sure Start', have shown the effectiveness of targeting areas of poverty to improve the welfare of the mother and her child.

However, it should also be recognised that those in higher social positions also have needs, especially in relation to emotional and mental health. Pregnancy can cause isolation for women who are used to being in employment, which may also result in loss of self-worth and status. Mental well-being promotion may include appropriate preparation for the realities of parenting and insurance that adequate physical and social support is available for the woman. High expectations of herself and the experience of labour may lead to feelings of disappointment or failure. Dependency on alcohol or drugs may also be a factor (NICE 2004).

TOTAL PREGNANCY CARE

Recognition of mental health disorders in pregnancy is an important role for the midwife, who may be the only health professional the woman will see consistently. It has been suggested that around 30% of pregnant women may experience depression with increased rates in those in lower socioeconomic groups (Bennett et al 2004). A recent study has demonstrated levels of self-reported depression may also be higher in the antenatal period than in the postnatal (Evans et al 2005). Within a holistic approach, it should be remembered that anything that may affect the well-being of the woman prior to pregnancy or in the antenatal period will subsequently have an effect during labour and in the postnatal continuum. Research has shown that antenatal psychological disturbance may have a long-term effect on a child's behaviour (O'Connor et al 2002). The same will apply for the care received during labour and the effect on the postnatal time. Issues in the postnatal period may also have an effect long into parenthood. Therefore, promotion of well-being should take place at all times for the potential effect it may have in the future on the well-being of the whole family.

Midwives on an individual basis may promote mental well-being in the people they encounter. Attitudes of caregivers have been shown to play a significant part in the happiness of women (Halldorsdottir & Karlsdottir 1996, Powell Kennedy 2000). Midwives should endeavour to be calm and relaxed and have a positive, caring attitude. It has also been suggested that to enable a therapeutic relationship, carers should demonstrate 'unconditional positive regard' as love (Stickley & Freshwater 2002), which has been linked to a spiritual focus of care (Hall 2001).

Good communication skills will also enhance well-being. For example, listening effectively, asking open questions, relaxed and open body language, not appearing rushed or in a hurry, use of appropriate touch and respect for the individual. These are all skills that may enable the woman to be empowered and to trust the midwife to be her advocate and support during a vulnerable time of her life.

The booking interview

The initial meeting between the midwife and pregnant woman is a significant time to introduce the woman to the maternity services. The assumption is that the midwife is interviewing the woman, however, independent midwives regard this time as the woman interviewing the midwife to see if she is the best one to care for her. This places the woman in control of the booking interview and thus empowers her.

The information required from the woman is often concentrated on the physical medical and obstetric history and family history. Issues in her family history of mental disorders should be noted and followed up for further information, as required. Questions regarding her experience of emotional disorder at the time of puberty and related to the menstrual cycle will alert the midwife to any issues that may arise in relation to hormone imbalance over the pregnancy or after the baby is born (Burt & Stein 2002). To ensure mental well-being, the midwife should also consider questions regarding the emotional state of the woman both currently in respect of the pregnancy and prior to the pregnancy occurring. Sometimes, unless women are asked directly, they may be reluctant to offer appropriate information. For example, if she has previously had a termination of pregnancy the midwife may be the first person she has spoken to since the event and she may need to deal with any negative feelings regarding her experience (Hall 1990). She may have also had previous miscarriages with feelings of grief, or this pregnancy may be the result of infertility treatment, which may have been a stressful experience (Harris 1994). Awareness of these issues should enable the midwife to support the woman more appropriately. Further evidence points to the potential of long-term mental disturbance, where women have experienced pregnancy loss combined with relationship difficulties and childhood abuse

(Bernazzani & Bifulco 2003). It should also not be assumed that this pregnancy is a welcome one and the midwife should be aware of any responses that may indicate the woman is unhappy. Awareness of the conditions in which the woman is living may indicate financial need and the support of social services may be offered. Issues relating to drug and alcohol dependency and domestic violence are explored later in the book, but the midwife should be alert to how these situations may impact on a woman's mental health.

Being aware of the spiritual need of the individual women is also appropriate. In North America, spiritual need is recognised as nursing diagnosis, with areas relating to both spiritual and religious beliefs (Table 3.1).

Table 3.1 Nursing diagnosis (North American Nursing Diagnosis Association)

Nursing diagnosis	Definition
Impaired religiosity	Impaired ability to exercise reliance on religious beliefs and/or participate in rituals of a particular faith tradition
Risk for impaired religiosity	At risk for an impaired ability to exercise reliance on religious beliefs and/or participate in rituals of a particular faith tradition
Readiness for enhanced religiosity	Ability to increase reliance on religious beliefs and/or participate in rituals of a particular faith tradition
Spiritual distress	Impaired ability to experience and integrate meaning and purpose in life through a person's connectedness with self, others, art, music, literature, nature or a power greater than oneself
Risk for spiritual distress	Risk for an impaired ability to experience and integrate meaning and purpose in life through a person's connectedness with self, others, art, music, literature, nature or a power greater than oneself
Readiness for enhanced spiritual well-being	Ability to experience and integrate meaning and purpose in life through a person's connectedness with self, others, art, music, literature, nature or a power greater than oneself

From: Burkhart (2005)

Though not specifically demonstrated as being appropriate for midwifery, these could be viewed as having application. Asking questions about what gives the woman meaning and purpose may demonstrate any values that she supports (Hall 2001); further it may be apparent from being in her home that she may have a religious faith of significance through artefacts or reading matter. As a midwife based in the community, it is also appropriate to have knowledge of the various religious communities or other support groups available to women. If signs of distress of a suspected spiritual nature are noted, suggesting to the women that they make contact with a local pastor or women's support group may provide the help they need.

Awareness of the social and physical needs of a woman is also important for her emotional health. There is evidence that shows the benefit of physical exercise to promote mental well-being (WHO 2005) and this may be a factor that could be introduced by midwives as part of their health promotion role.

Antenatal care

Throughout the antenatal period, the midwife should be aware of times when the woman may be vulnerable to emotional stress. For example, physical illness in pregnancy, such as hyperemesis gravidarum or anaemia, may lead to severe tiredness and to poor mental adjustment (Cantwell & Cox 2003). She may also experience spiritual distress and feel unable to pray or participate in her usual religious or spiritual rituals. The woman may be vulnerable to distress when leaving her place of employment for maternity leave. Emotional reactions may be experienced through broken relationships (Richards et al 1997); however, some women may feel better after broken relationships that have been abusive or stressful. Financial difficulties may also have an impact on the mental health of the woman and her family (Nettleton & Burrows 1998). The midwife should be aware of emotional events, e.g. if the woman experiences the loss of a close family member or moves area during the pregnancy and these are times when she will be susceptible to a grief reaction. This may also be experienced at the anniversary of the time a previous lost baby, either by miscarriage, termination or stillbirth, would have been born (Franco et al 1989, Hall 1990, Kersting et al 2005, Korenromp et al 2005). Though grief is a normal reaction to loss, the midwife should be aware of the reaction being excessive. Recognition of the effects of fear upon the emotional state of the woman is also important. Hofberg & Ward (2004) describe different levels of fear:

- Primary tocophobia: where the woman has never experienced pregnancy
- Secondary tocophobia: usually as a result of a previous traumatic birth
- Secondary depressive illness in the antenatal period.

Such fears, if not addressed may lead to requests for a caesarean delivery (Ryding 1993).

If the booking questions have been asked appropriately, then previous personal psychiatric disorders may have already arisen. However, distinction should be made between manifestations of previous mental health disorders and specific disorders as a result of the present pregnancy. These are discussed in more depth later in the book, but midwives need to be aware of conditions that will require referral to other agencies for diagnosis and potential treatment.

Labour

The time of giving birth is a significantly powerful and potentially stressful time where the emotional state of the woman and her partner are in a particularly vulnerable place. The midwife has responsibility to promote not only physical safety but also emotional safety. At this time, the physical/emotional/spiritual experiences are close and deeply impacting on each other. The emotional relationship between birth and death is close. The experiences that take place at this time may have a long-lasting effect upon the woman, her partner and the unborn baby (Waldenstrom 2004). The recognition of this as important is significant for the carers who are both there providing care during the labour and during the planning phase. The choices that women make about where she has her baby, who is there facilitating it and her expectations about what will happen, will have significance and meaning to her. The removal of that choice, or a change to her expectations may cause distress. It is important for caregivers to recognise this stress and provide support to the woman to help in her acceptance of the situation. The need to care appropriately and for women to remain in control is also important (Green & Baston 2003, Halldorsdottir & Karlsdottir 1996). The disempowerment of women through choice being removed or through coercion may subsequently be damaging. The midwife's role in empowering a woman through her labour is significant in promoting well-being (Halldorsdottir & Karlsdottir 1996). The midwife's belief in the woman's ability to give birth is important as is the ability to ensure the woman still feels empowered and part of her labour, in situations where there is need for intervention. The impact of a labour that is disempowering is long term and can lead to fears, anxiety and post-traumatic stress disorder. Suggestions that postnatal debriefing is valuable for certain groups of women has been demonstrated (Gamble et al 2005) but it may be more appropriate to examine the care and practices around the time of labour that lead to the initial distress. Recognition of the impact of antenatal issues or of the effect of previous birth experiences should not be discounted.

Case study

Powell Kennedy & MacDonald (2002) record the story told by a midwife of a woman's experience of birth. In this situation, the woman, at the end of the birth, became unresponsive despite her showing no physical signs of collapse. Some 25 min later the woman opened her eyes and began responding. The following day, the midwife went to see her and gently questioned her about the birth. The woman revealed that the experience had been bad and she had experienced leaving her body and watching the midwife from the ceiling. She had eventually returned to her body to 'come back for my baby'. Furthermore, she revealed a previous traumatic history of birth and described a 'heavy sadness'. The gentle probing by the midwife enabled the woman to express her need and mental therapies were offered and accepted. The story is completed with the woman having a further positive birth. The authors conclude:

'Not all women, when asked, will disclose a family history of traumas or abuse, and many in fact cannot remember. Even though this may happen it is still essential that the questions are asked and that an environment that is safe, caring and accepting is created. The stage is then set for her to trust in the future'.

(Powell Kennedy & MacDonald 2002)

In the circumstances of birth, the woman must feel safe and secure and should have privacy (Odent 1994). The provision of a more home-like birth environment may have an effect on women's fears and anxieties and promote their well-being (Newburn 2006).

During labour, the ability to cope with pain should be gauged. The relationship between fear and anxiety levels and the ability to cope with pain may have a significant effect. Ideally, the midwife should, during the antenatal period, have learnt how the woman copes with issues of pain. If she is used to turning immediately to pharmacological methods for dealing with a headache, for example, she is likely to do the same when dealing with birth. Grantly Dick-Read's (2004) work on fear related to tension and pain may be appropriate to some women in order to manage their experience of labour. Others have shown the spiritual value of psychologically expressing pain as a positive emotion (Gaskin 2002). Some women may turn to the use of complementary therapies to help them through labour, however it should be ensured that in an holistic sense the right therapies are chosen for the particular individual (Wickham 2006). Changing the environment around birth as well as increasing the use of massage techniques may also have an effect (Haines & Kimber 2005a,b).

The promotion of skin-to-skin contact with the baby after birth for a significant uninterrupted time may promote increased well-being as the family unit come to terms with the arrival of the new person in their life (Kennell & McGrath 2005), as well as the promotion of breastfeeding (Carfoot et al 2003). Enabling an environment where this can take place in a busy birthing suite is a challenge but has the potential of positive long-term effects for the woman and her baby.

Postnatal

In the early days after having a baby, women are very vulnerable to the changes that are taking place physically, emotionally, spiritually and socially. The alteration in the hormonal state of women will not affect each woman emotionally in the same way and there may be some relationship to how she was affected in relation to menstruation (Burt & Stein 2002). However, it is common for a woman to experience emotional feelings following the birth of her baby. These issues will be explored in greater depth later in this book, however there is much that midwives can do to promote the emotional well-being of women. Current postnatal care in UK hospitals has been fragmented with women complaining of feeling unsupported in relation to practical care as well as emotionally. Community postnatal care has been shown to have a positive effect on women's emotional well-being (MacArthur et al 2002). The following list identifies the risk factors for those who may be most at risk of postnatal depression (Powell Kennedy et al 2002):

- Prior history of depressive illness before or during pregnancy
- Child care stress
- Life stress
- Lack of social support
- Prenatal anxiety
- Maternity blues
- Marital dissatisfaction
- Low self-esteem
- Low socioeconomic status
- Single
- Unplanned or undesired pregnancy.

Those women who may have become pregnant through reproductive technologies may have more difficulty in adjustment. It is suggested that it may be related to no longer needing to 'perform sexually on command' or due to the loss of the intensive connections with medical carers (Burt & Hendrick 1997:100–101). Being able to identify those women most at risk means that midwives can facilitate better support during the early postnatal period and beyond.

Sleep deprivation is a key factor affecting both women and their partners (Bozoky & Corwin 2002). Altered patterns in REM sleep in the early postnatal period lead to greater fatigue (Lee et al 2000). The disturbance may further be increased where the woman's labour has been long and has resulted in a traumatic or surgical birth. Sherr (1995:200–201) has suggested that busy postnatal wards are not the ideal environments for women to have the opportunity for restful sleep. Adapting practices on postnatal wards to promote a restful environment and promote sleep for women is important and should be put into place. These can include:

- Dropping 'routine' and task orientated practices to fit in with shifts
- Lowering of noise levels generally through wearing soft shoes, lowering conversation levels, reducing levels of television or radio noise

- Mending squeaking equipment
- Reducing levels of light at night
- Communicating with visitors through leaflets or verbally to explain importance of rest (Hall 2005).

Practical support for women in the postnatal period is normal practice in other countries (van Teijlingen 1993) and this may be increased through the use of maternity care assistants in the community (Lindsay 2004). Recognition that women need support is important and it should not be assumed that those from higher social groups need less support (NICE 2004). Promoting long-term well-being may be through encouraging women to look after their health, e.g. encouraging exercise and healthy eating practices, which will assist in their physical well-being but also has been shown to promote mental well-being (Hawkins 2005a). Promoting the woman's mothering skills and helping her to find meaning and purpose in the event will promote her spiritual well-being (Hall 2001). Encouraging the woman to touch and massage her baby may benefit all women and their babies as it has been shown to help those who have signs of postnatal depressive illness (Onozawa et al 2001). Midwives are in an important position to recognise the signs of mental disturbance in partners. The link between partner depression and maternal depression is recognised (Goodman 2004) and this may have a further effect on the well-being of the infant (Ramchandani et al 2005). Therefore, community midwifery may work in partnership with others in the primary care team to provide support to families where mental health needs are apparent.

CONCLUSION

The aim of this chapter has been to explore ways in which mental well-being may be promoted in relation to women and childbirth issues. It has been demonstrated that midwives and other carers can examine the current services and create environments where it is conducive to support and enable women in their adjustment to being mothers. Recognition of the holistic nature of people will also enable a different approach to care that will foster well-being in all aspects of their lives.

References

Antonovsky A 1993 The implications of salutogenesis: an outsider's view. In: Turnbull AP, Patterson JM, Behr SG et al (eds) Cognitive coping: families and disability. Brookes, Baltimore

Bastard J, Tiran D 2006 Aromatherapy and massage for antenatal anxiety: its effect on the fetus. Complementary Therapies in Clinical Practice 12(1): 48–54

Bennett H A, Einarson A, Taddio A et al 2004 Depression during pregnancy: Overview of clinical factors. Clinical Drug Investigation 24(30):157–179

Bernazzani O, Bifulco A 2003 Motherhood as a vulnerability factor in major depression: the role of negative pregnancy experiences. Social Science and Medicine 56(6):1249–1260

Bozoky I, Corwin E J 2002 Fatigue as a predictor of postpartum depression. Journal of Obstetric, Gynecologic, and Neonatal Nursing 31:436–443

Brimblecombe N R 2004 The changing relationship between mental health nurses and psychiatrists in the United Kingdom. Journal of Advanced Nursing 49(4):344–353

Burkhart L 2005 Documenting spiritual care. Journal of Christian Nursing 22(1):6–12

Burt V K, Hendrick V C 1997 Concise guide to women's mental health. American Psychiatric Press, Washington

Burt V K, Stein K 2002 Epidemiology of depression throughout the female life cycle. Journal of Clinical Psychiatry 63(suppl 7):9–15

Cantwell R, Cox J L 2003 Psychiatric disorders in pregnancy and the puerperium. Current Obstetrics and Gynecology 13:7–13

Carfoot S, Williamson P, Dickson R 2003 Successful breastfeeding: a systematic review of randomised controlled trials evaluating the effect of mother/infant skin-to-skin care. Midwifery 19:148–155

Commission of the European Communities (CEC) 2005 Green paper: Improving the mental health of the population. Towards a strategy on mental health for the European Union Brussels, 484 final. Online. Available: http://www.eu-oplysningen.dk/upload/application/pdf/e752d81a/20050484.pdf 14 Oct 2005

Department of Health (DoH) 1993 Changing childbirth. HMSO, London

Department of Health (DoH) 1999 National service framework for mental health. Modern standards & service models. Department of Health, London

Department of Health (DoH) 2004 National service framework for children, young people and maternity services: maternity services. Department of Health, London

Department of Health (DoH) 2005 Delivering, choosing health: making healthier choices easier. Department of Health, London

Department of Health (DoH) 2006 Our health, our care, our say: a new direction for community services. Department of Health, London

Dick-Read G 2004 Childbirth without fear: the principles and practice of natural childbirth. Pinter & Martin, London

Dombeck M-T 1996 Chaos and self-organization as a consequence of spiritual disequilibrium. Clinical Nurse Specialist 10(2):69–73

Evans J, Heron J, Francomb H et al 2005 Cohort study of depressed mood during pregnancy and after childbirth. British Medical Journal 323:257–260

Flint C, Poulangeris P 1986 The 'Know your midwife' report. Available: 49 Peckarman's Wood, Sydenham Hill, London SE26 6RZ, UK

Franco K, Campbell N, Tamburrino M et al 1989 Anniversary reactions and due date responses following abortion. Psychotherapy and Psychosomatics 52(1):151–154

Galea S, Ahern J, Rudenstine S et al 2005 Urban built environment and depression: a multilevel analysis. Journal of Epidemiology and Community Health 59(10):822–827

Gamble J, Creedy D, Moyle W et al 2005 Effectiveness of a counseling intervention after a traumatic childbirth: a randomized controlled trial. Birth 32(1):11–19

Gaskin I M 2002 Spiritual midwifery, 3rd edn. Book Publishing Company, Summertown, Tennessee

Goodman J 2004 Paternal postpartum depression, its relationship to maternal postpartum depression, and implications for family health. Journal of Advanced Nursing 45:26–35

Goodwin I, Holmes G, Newnes C et al 2000 A qualitative analysis of the views of in-patient mental health service users. Journal of Mental Health 8:43–54

Green J M, Baston H A 2003 Feeling in control during labor: concepts, correlates, and consequences. Birth 30(4):235–249

Haines A, Kimber L 2005a Improving the birthing environment (Part 1). Practising Midwife 8(1):18–20

Haines A, Kimber L 2005b Improving the birthing environment (Part 2). Practising Midwife 8(2):25–27

Hall J 1990 A hard decision – Psychological effects of termination on subsequent pregnancy. Nursing Times 28(47):32–35

Hall J 2001 Midwifery, mind and spirit: emerging issues of care. Books for Midwives, Oxford

Hall J 2005 Postnatal emotional well-being. The Practising Midwife 8(4):35–40

Halldorsdottir S, Karlsdottir S I 1996 Empowerment or discouragement: women's experience of caring and uncaring encounters during childbirth. Healthcare for Women International 17:361–379

Harris R E 1994 The process of infertility. In: Field PA, Marck PB (eds) Uncertain motherhood: negotiating the risks of the childbearing years. SAGE, London

Hawkins J 2005a Alternative treatments for depression: Exercise and 'wake' therapy. Journal of Holistic Healthcare 2(2):9–16

Hawkins J 2005b Alternative treatments for depression: light and St John's Wort. Journal of Holistic Healthcare 2(4):19–26

Health Education Authority (1997) Mental health promotion: a quality framework. Health Education Authority, London

Hofberg K, Ward M R 2004 Fear of childbirth, tocophobia and mental health in mothers: the obstetric-psychiatric interface. Clinical Obstetrics and Gynaecology 47(3):527–534

Kaufmann T 2002 Midwifery and public health. MIDIRS Midwifery Digest 12(suppl 1):S23–S26

Kennell J, McGrath S 2005 Starting the process of mother-infant bonding. Acta Paediatrica 94(6):775–777

Kersting A, Dorsch M, Kreulich C et al 2005 Trauma and grief 2–7 years after termination of pregnancy because of fetal anomalies – a pilot study. Journal of Psychosomatic Obstetrics and Gynecology 26(1):9–14

Kirkham M 2003 Birth centres as an enabling culture. In: Kirkham M (ed.) Birth centres: a social model for maternity care. Books for Midwives, Oxford

Koenig H G 2005 Faith and mental health: religious resources for healing. Templeton Foundation Press, London

Korenromp M J, Christiaens G C, van den Bout J et al 2005 Long-term psychological consequences of pregnancy termination for fetal abnormality: a cross-sectional study. Prenatal Diagnosis 25(3):253–260

Lee K A, Zaffke M E, McEnany G 2000 Parity and sleep patterns during and after pregnancy. Obstetrics and Gynaecology 95:14–18

Lindsay P 2004 Introduction of maternity care assistants. British Journal of Midwifery 12(10):650–653

MacArthur C, Winter H, Bick D, et al 2002 Effects of redesigned community postnatal care on womens' health 4 months after birth: a cluster randomised controlled trial. The Lancet 359(9304):378–385

McCourt C, Page L, Hewison J et al 1998 Evaluation of one-to-one midwifery. Women's responses to care. Birth 25(2):73–80

Morris K 2002 Does art work in mental health? The Lancet 360(9339):1104

Newburn M 2006 Curtains for the old delivery suite. The Practising Midwife 9(1):12–14

National Institute for Clinical Excellence (NICE), The Scottish Executive Health Department and The Department of Health Social Services and Public Safety: Northern Ireland 2004 The confidential enquiries into maternal deaths in the United Kingdom. Why mothers die 2000–2002. RCOG, London

Nettleton S, Burrows R 1998 Mortgage debt, insecure home ownership and health: an exploratory analysis. Sociology of Health and Illness 20(5):731–753

O'Connor T G, Heron J, Glover V, The Alspac study team 2002 Antenatal anxiety predicts child behavioural/emotional problems independently of postnatal depression. Journal of the American Academy of Child and Adolescent Psychiatry 41(12):1470–1477

Odent M 1994 Birth reborn: what childbirth should be. Souvenir Press, London

Onozawa K, Glover V, Adams D et al 2001 Infant massage improves mother-infant interaction for mothers with postnatal depression. Journal of Affective Disorders 63(1–3):201–207

Peters D 2005 Holism, mental health and mental wealth. Journal of Holistic Healthcare 2(4):2

Poulton R, Caspi A, Milne B J et al 2002 Association between children's experience of socioeconomic disadvantage and adult health: a life-course study. The Lancet 360(9346):1640–1645

Powell Kennedy H 2000 A model of exemplary midwifery practice: results of a Delphi study. Journal of Midwifery and Women's Health 45(1):4–19

Powell Kennedy H, MacDonald E L 2002 'Altered consciousness' during childbirth: potential clues to post-traumatic stress disorder. Journal of Midwifery and Women's Health 74(5):380–382

Powell Kennedy H, Tatano Beck C, Watson Driscoll J 2002 A light in the fog: caring for women with postpartum depression. Journal of Midwifery and Women's Health 47(5):318–327

Pullon S, Fry B 2005 Interprofessional postgraduate education in primary healthcare: Is it making a difference? Journal of Interprofessional Care 19(6):569–578

Ramchandani P, Stein A, Evans J et al 2005 Paternal depression in the postnatal period and child development: a prospective population study. The Lancet 365(9478):2201–2205

Richards M, Hardy R, Wadsworth G 1997 The effects of divorce and separation on mental health in a national UK birth cohort. Psychological Medicine 27:1121–1128

Robinson M, Cottrell D 2005 Health professionals in multi-disciplinary and multi-agency teams: Changing professional practice. Journal of Interprofessional Care 19(6):547–560

Royal College of Midwives (RCM) 2001 The midwife's role in public health. RCM position paper 24. Online. Available: http://www.rcm.org.uk/info/pages/introduction.php?id=4 12 Jan 2006

Royal College of Midwives (RCM) 2002 What is salutogenesis? Online. Available: http://www.rcm.org.uk/data/info_centre/data/virtual_institute_salutogenesis.htm 12 Jan 2006

Ryding E L 1993 Investigations of 33 women who demanded a caesarean section for personal reasons. Acta Obstetricia Gynecologica Scandinavica 72:280–285

Sainsbury's Centre for mental health 2006 The future of mental health: a vision for 2015. Online. Available: http://www.scmh.org.uk/80256FBD004F6342/vWeb/pcKHAL6KPF25 11 Apr 2006

Sherr L 1995 The psychology of pregnancy and childbirth. Blackwell Science, Oxford

Skapinakis P, Lewis G, Araya R et al 2005 Mental health inequalities in Wales, UK: multi-level investigation of the effect of area deprivation. British Journal of Psychiatry 186:417–422

Stickley T, Freshwater D 2002 The art of loving and the therapeutic relationship. Nursing Inquiry 9(4):250–256

Swinton J 2001 Spirituality and mental healthcare. Jessica Kingsley, London

Timms P 2003 Coping with a physical illness. Royal College of Psychiatrists, London

van Teijlingen E R 1993 Maternity home-care assistants: a unique occupation. In: Abraham-Van der mark E (ed.) Successful home birth and midwifery: the Dutch model. Bergin & Garvey, London

Waldenstrom U 2004 Why do some women change their opinion about childbirth over time? Birth 31(2):102–107

Waller S, Finn H 2004 Enhancing the healing environment: a guide for NHS trusts. King's Fund, London

WHO 1948 Preamble to the constitution of the World Health Organization as adopted by the International Health Conference, New York, 19–22 June, 1946; signed on 22 July 1946 by the representatives of 61 States (Official Records of the World Health Organization, No. 2: 100) and entered into force on 7 April 1948. Online. Available: http://www.who.int/about/definition/en 12 Sept 2005

WHO 2000 Women and mental health. Online. Available: http://www.who.int/mediacentre/factsheets/fs248/en/print.html 12 Sept 2005

WHO 2001 A public health approach to mental health. Online. Available: http://www.who.int/whr/2001/chapter1/en/index1.html 12 Sept 2005

WHO 2004 Strategies to improving empowerment through advocacy. Online. Available: www.who.dk/document/mnh/ebrief05.pdf 20 Sept 2005

WHO 2005 Why move for health. Online. Available: http://www.who.int/moveforhealth/en/ 9 Feb 2005

Wickham S 2006 Holistic tensions: is West really best? The Practising Midwife 9(3):4–5

Chapter **4**

The development and organisation of contemporary mental health services

Anthony Harrison

INTRODUCTION

While mental healthcare had been characterised by marked change and development throughout the late twentieth and early twenty-first centuries, it can also be said that much has remained the same. Historically, mental healthcare has been seen as the 'Cinderella' service when compared with other aspects of healthcare; something which remains a contemporary issue for mental health providers, workers, service users and carers. Although it is estimated that mental health problems in the UK cost £7.7 billion each year, the proportion of money spent on mental health services is significantly less than other areas of health service spending (King's Fund 2005). It is against this background that professionals, carers, non-statutory agencies and volunteers struggle to provide effective mental healthcare across all age ranges.

This chapter provides an overview of the development and organisation of contemporary mental healthcare in the UK. It will describe the historical influences on the delivery of mental health services, the growth of the service user and carer movements and finally provides a commentary on the role of non-psychiatric staff, such as midwives and health visitors, in the provision of mental healthcare.

HISTORICAL PERSPECTIVES

Mental illness and distress has existed since primitive times and society's understanding and interpretation of these concepts need to be seen in their historical context. In every culture there is an awareness of 'psychological difference' with specific explanations and approaches to the understanding, care, treatment and social management of individuals who are mentally distressed, anxious, vulnerable and frightened (Pilgrim & Rogers 1999). Early interpretations of mental distress, often manifesting in the form of bizarre, strange or 'abnormal' behaviour, were largely influenced by religious and spiritual beliefs, as individuals were thought to be possessed by demons and evil spirits. The societal response to such distress was to drive out the evil spirits through religious rituals, magic and reincarnation (Hayes 2000) and sufferers were largely rejected and excluded from the mainstream group or community.

These early views persisted through the Middle Ages and into the late seventeenth and early eighteenth centuries, with individuals who were considered to be mentally disturbed either being locked away in prison or simply left to roam the streets and countryside. Certain religious orders demonstrated compassion and early forms of caring for people who were mentally ill were undertaken in a few monasteries and convents (Nolan 1993). A religious retreat was opened at York in 1792 by the Quaker William Tuke and was established on the principle of 'moral treatment', whereby punishment, cruelty and degradation were replaced by social, occupational and educational activities (Norman & Ryrie 2004). The Bethlam Royal Hospital in London had been established in 1247 and for centuries was one of a very few hospitals in Europe that cared for people who were considered insane. Patients were admitted from all over the country. The main local alternatives which were to appear later were private madhouses, which flourished from the eighteenth century onwards, and the county asylums of the nineteenth century.

From the late seventeenth century, the biomedical model came to dominate society's understanding of health and illness, and it was developments in the understanding of anatomy and physiology, largely through the study of the body post-mortem, that led to rapid advances in treatments for physical illnesses (Turp 2001). The French philosopher René Descartes developed the idea that the mind and body are two separate entities, believing that because the body is a material object, it can be understood through scientific study and physical examination, but that the mind is of a higher order and can therefore only be understood through introspection. This dualistic perspective, characterised by the theoretical separation of mind and body paved the way for the development of psychological models in the understanding of mental distress, and focused on the secular philosophical analysis and interpretation of mental phenomena. However, it was not until the twentieth century that specific psychological models and therapies influenced mainstream approaches to the care and treatment of people who were mentally unwell.

The nineteenth century saw the establishment and proliferation of large institutions across the UK for the treatment of the insane, with each county having its own asylum, many of which catered for well over 1000 inmates. Most of these institutions were built from the mid-1850s to the 1920s and at their peak provided inpatient care for over 140 000 individuals (Ford 2004). The work in these asylums was organised and delivered on an institutionalised basis, with the focus of much staff activity on the smooth running of the asylum, with its hierarchical structures, task-orientated activities and physical security and containment. Some viewed the establishment of the asylums as an example of a massive Victorian experiment in social engineering (Barcan & Glazier 1997).

During the twentieth century, dominant views began to shift; the interwar years, nursing registration, developing schools of psychological thought, such as Freudian analytical theories, the establishment of the national health service (NHS) and the development of pharmacological treatments such as major tranquilisers, all influenced the change from incarceration to one of care, treatment and cure (Norman & Ryrie 2004). By the late 1950s there was a growing movement away from the concept of institutionalised hospital care to that of community-orientated care for people suffering from mental illness. A number of factors have been cited as influencing the development of community-based mental health services (Norman & Ryrie 2004) and include the following:

- Overcrowding of mental hospitals
- Dilapidated state of buildings and poor physical environment of the Victorian asylums
- Mental health legislation, in particular the 1959 Mental Health Act, that stressed the importance of community involvement in psychiatric care
- Shift in the power base from the former superintendent physicians to the developing role of independent psychiatrists, paving the way for more individually focused and case managed care, as opposed to institutionalised asylum-based regimes
- Discovery of new psychiatric medications, such as antipsychotics (also known as major tranquilisers) and antidepressants, that for the first time were able to control the worst excesses of

behavioural disturbance and in some instances provide an effective treatment for conditions such as depression.

Institutionalised, hospital-based care came under increasing scrutiny in the 1960s, with the simultaneous growth in what became known as the 'anti-psychiatry' movement. Prominent individuals in this movement included the author Goffman (1961), who questioned orthodox approaches to understanding mental distress as promulgated by the psychiatric professionals and services of the day. He challenged this philosophical position and the notion that mental distress should sit within a biomedical paradigm. Instead he emphasised how psychiatry, as practised at the time, was largely used as a means of social control and that the imprecise nature of diagnostic reasoning meant that the understanding and responses to mental distress as a society and as professionals was far from comprehensive (Nolan 1993). Goffman's seminal work in 1961 on the nature and effects of the asylum on the individual did more than most contemporary criticism to question and challenge the prevailing orthodoxy. This was followed by a number of high profile cases of abuse of patients by staff at a number of psychiatric hospitals in the UK and the concomitant public unease about existing psychiatric institutions (Yorkshire Television 1979). Prior to the establishment of the NHS in 1948, the government had already recognised the shortcomings of the way in which mental healthcare was organised, citing the wide variation in policy and practice across the country, poorly coordinated mental health nurse training and staff that were often as institutionalised as the patients (MoH 1945).

During the 1970s and 1980s there was an accelerated closure programme of the large institutions, with the establishment of smaller mental health units as part of general hospitals and within local communities. Community care initially followed an outreach model with psychiatric nurses, who continued to be hospital-based, providing a service to individual patients either in their own homes or by visiting community units, hostels and nursing homes. Community mental health teams (CMHTs) were developed in the 1980s, consisting of a range of professions such as medicine, nursing, psychology, occupational therapy and social work, all within one team. For the most part, such teams now provide the main focus for the provision of mental healthcare within local communities, undertaking an assessment and liaison service to primary care, as well as providing a range of community-based treatment options as alternatives to hospital admission.

ORGANISATION AND DELIVERY OF CONTEMPORARY MENTAL HEALTHCARE

National policy has shaped the provision of mental health services since psychiatric care was incorporated into the NHS in 1948. The focus of central health policies since the 1950s has been on the establishment and strengthening of community-based services, with an expansion in professional roles located in a range of primary and secondary care settings. Mental healthcare is now delivered across the whole spectrum of health and social care services and by a range of providers, and is commissioned by primary care trusts (PCTs) on behalf of their local population (Table 4.1). In England, strategic health authorities (SHAs) provide a monitoring and quality assurance function in terms of ensuring that national policy and central directives are delivered. Since 1997, the organisation and delivery

Table 4.1 Overview of organisations providing mental health services

Sector	Examples and descriptions
Specialist NHS trusts	Full range of mental health services within a defined area
	Includes CMHTs, inpatient services, specialist services, e.g. psychotherapy, mental health liaison with the general hospital, court diversion, prison in-reach, etc.
Local authority social service departments	May provide services in collaboration and in conjunction with NHS trusts
	Offer services such as the provision of approved social workers (ASWs), community support teams, day centres, nursing and residential homes
Profit-making private sector	May provide a range of specialist services, including in-patient care, psychotherapy and counselling services, low and medium secure forensic services
Non-profit-making voluntary sector	May provide a range of specialist and non-specialist services, including support groups, day care, advocacy services, befriending and service user involvement.
	Organisations include MIND, Rethink, The Samaritans, Age Concern

(See Bloom 2006, NICE 2004, Read et al 2003, Stillman-Lowe 1997)

of mental health services has been informed by the following government initiatives:

- Reforms to the commissioning and funding of health and social care, and the publication of various reports, standards for good practice and other policy initiatives (Table 4.2)
- Publication of specific National Service Frameworks (NSFs), each providing a template for the organisational delivery and standards relating to specific groups or health conditions, e.g. NSFs for mental health (DoH 1999a) and older people (DoH 2001)
- Establishment of the National Institute for Clinical Excellence (NICE) in 2000
- Establishment of the National Institute for Mental Health in England (NIMHE) in 2001
- Establishment of the National Patient Safety Agency (NPSA) in 2001
- Establishment of the Healthcare Commission (replacing the Commission for Health Improvement) in 2004.

The diverse causes and contributory factors to mental health problems, alongside the various presentations of mental distress, mean that the majority of mental healthcare is delivered by non-statutory services; factors such as meaningful occupation and employment, safe relationships, appropriate accommodation and housing, educational opportunities, and financial security will all influence a person's mental health. When an individual is in need of formal mental healthcare this may be accessed and delivered by a variety of means, and is often provided by non-mental health staff. The role of practice nurses, midwives, health visitors and general practitioners in the provision of mental healthcare is well recognised and there is now a growing emphasis on mental health skills and interventions being provided in non-psychiatric settings and by non-mental health services (Harrison & Hart 2006). Added to this is the diverse nature and wide variation in the way that local mental health services are planned, commissioned and provided, which despite the growth in policy and practice guidance, means that it is not possible to provide a definitive outline of the organisation of mental healthcare within a particular geographical area. However, all services are expected to conform to the delivery targets and quality milestones identified within the relevant NSFs, in particular those relating to mental health and children, young people and maternity services. Other NSFs, such as those for cancer and older people are also of relevance, as are the clinical guidelines issued by

Table 4.2   Selected summary of policies, reports and guidance shaping the delivery of mental health services since 1997

Policy/report	Commentary
Modernising Mental Health Services (DoH 1998)	The first comprehensive statement regarding the future direction of mental health policy for over 20 years
	Pledged £700 million to improve mental health services, including better outreach services, improved access to newer antipsychotic medication and 24-h crisis teams
NSF for Mental Health (DoH 1999a)	Aimed at eliminating the wide variations in standards of mental healthcare
	Focuses on the mental health needs of adults of working age, up to 65 years
	Identifies seven key standards based on current evidence and outlining examples of good practice
	Highlights the incidence of mental illness in the postnatal period and emphasises the increased risk of suicide in mothers following childbirth
Saving Lives: Our Healthier Nation (DoH 1999b)	Identifies the need to reduce the national suicide rate by one-fifth (20%) by 2010
	Outlines a vision for improving the mental health of the population through mental health promotion strategies
The NHS Plan (DoH 2000)	£300 million to 'fast forward' the targets identified in the mental health NSF (DoH 2000)
	Sets targets for specific services and new teams, including gateway mental health workers within primary care, establishment of assertive outreach, crisis resolution and women-only services, prison mental healthcare, secure accommodation for people with personality disorder and the provision of respite for carers
NSF for Older People (DoH 2001)	Identifies eight standards for effective health and social care of older people
	Standard 7 focuses on mental health and emphasises the need to collaborate across services

Table 4.2 Continued

Policy/report	Commentary
National Suicide Prevention Strategy for England (DoH 2002)	Provides detailed policy guidance as a means of achieving the suicide reduction target identified in Saving Lives: Our Healthier Nation (DoH 1999a) Identified six goals ranging from encouraging the sensitive reporting of suicide in the media, the promotion of suicide research and improved primary and secondary suicide prevention
Mainstreaming Gender and Women's Mental Health (DoH 2003a)	Identifies broad guidance to support the planning and delivery of mental health services to ensure that women feel better served by the mental healthcare system Focuses on a wide range of clinical and practice areas, including perinatal mental health, sexual and relationship abuse/violence and substance misuse
Essence of Care (DoH 2003b)	Originally launched in 2001, focuses on the fundamental aspects of the service user's/patient's experience Addresses issues such as privacy and dignity, record keeping and the safety of people who have mental health needs but who are being cared for in non-mental-health settings by non-mental-health staff
Antenatal Care: Routine Care for the Healthy Pregnant Woman (National Collaborating Centre for Women's and Children's Health 2003)	Aims to inform best practice in clinical care for all pregnancies in healthy women. Provides evidence-based advice regarding psychological responses to pregnancy and childbirth, psychiatric disorders domestic/relationship violence and mental health promotion
NSF for Children, Young People and Maternity Services (DoH 2004)	A 10-year programme consisting of core standards (those that all NHS services have to meet) and developmental standards (those that should be targets for service and clinical improvement)

Table 4.2   Continued

Policy/report	Commentary
	The five core standards focus on health (including mental health) promotion, supporting parenting, family-centred services, growing into adulthood and safeguarding children and young people
Why Mothers Die 2000–2002. Confidential Enquires into Maternal and Child Health (NICE et al 2004)	Reports on the causes, nature and trends in maternal deaths
	Identifies mental health problems as a significant cause of morbidity and mortality – the largest cause of maternal deaths overall was psychiatric illness

the National Institute for Clinical Excellence (NICE). Core standards for the provision of mental healthcare, as set out in the mental health NSF will inform the delivery of local services and are summarised in Box 4.1.

Box 4.1 Summary of the core standards within the NSF for mental health

- All health and social care services should take positive steps to promote mental health, combat discrimination and challenge stigmatising attitudes
- Primary care staff should provide effective and timely assessment of mental health need
- 24-h access to services for people with a mental health problem
- Access to specialist services for people with a known mental health problem within the framework of the Care Programme Approach (CPA)
- Carers to have their needs assessed
- Lead organisations to actively address the target of suicide reduction (Table 4.2).

(DoH 1999a)

Although there has been a significant increase in the range of community-based mental health services since 2000, within the majority of health communities, the CMHT continues to be a major focus for the provision of mental healthcare. CMHTs provide the first contact point for the majority of individuals who require referral on for a specialist mental health assessment, and have a role in accepting referrals from primary care, in-patient mental health services, secondary care services and non-mental health teams, such as police, probation and the non-statutory sector (Onyett & Smith 1998). Team structures and systems vary, but CMHTs have a range of professionals based within them and provide an assessment, advice, liaison, intervention, education and case management role for those individuals referred and accepted onto a team member's case load. For most people who are suffering from a severe and enduring mental illness, the CMHT will provide a case management, care management and individual intervention role, working within the framework of the Care Programme Approach (CPA) (DoH 1990). The CPA requires that an individual practitioner, often a community mental health nurse (CMHN) or social worker, undertake the role of care coordinator, overseeing the planning and coordination of care, and taking responsibility for ensuring effective communication between the service user, carer(s) and other statutory and non-statutory services that may be providing input into the person's total package of care. The CMHT care coordinator will also act as a link between the various parts of the mental health service, in particular if the service user is receiving care from more than one team within a local area (Box 4.2).

The processes and mechanisms involved in referral, assessment, care and treatment planning, evaluation and care coordination can appear complex to those unfamiliar with the provision of mental health services. Each process will vary slightly according to the way local services have been set up and the resources allocated to the various teams and roles. However, the principles of service delivery should be consistent throughout the NHS (Table 4.3).

SERVICE USER AND CARER INVOLVEMENT AND PARTICIPATION

The mental health service user movement has developed a profile and visibility as a result of the challenges to dominant philosophical assumptions about mental illness, mental distress and social exclusion. The service user movement is underpinned by funda-

Box 4.2 The range of statutory mental health teams within a typical health community

- Primary care mental health gateway workers: providing a service for individuals with less severe mental health problems (e.g. mild to moderate depression and anxiety) within the primary care setting and in collaboration with GPs, practice nurses, midwives and health visitors
- Child and adolescent mental health services (CAMHS): specialist community and residential mental healthcare for children, families and young people
- Community mental health teams (CMHTs): often providing a single point of entry into local mental health services for those referred from both primary and secondary care
- In-patient psychiatric services: hospital-based
- Crisis services: providing an urgent assessment and intervention service for individuals/families experiencing a mental health crisis or psychiatric emergency
- Assertive outreach teams: working with a relatively small caseload of individuals and families who are suffering from severe mental illness and who are at risk of disengagement with treatment and care because of the nature of their mental health problem
- Intensive home treatment teams: provide an alternative to hospital admission and facilitate early discharge from inpatient units
- Mental health liaison teams: general hospital-based teams providing a mental health assessment and intervention service to the acute hospital
- Court diversion and youth offending teams: provide a service aimed at identifying those people within the court and criminal justice systems who are suffering from mental illness, and at ensuring they receive mental healthcare if needed.

mental questions regarding the role of medicine in the form of psychiatry, the role of professionals in responding to mental distress and the growth in consumerism generally throughout society and the NHS in particular. Individuals who use mental health services are in many instances actively engaged in recounting their experiences of services and in offering their expertise in the planning,

Table 4.3   Overview of effective care coordination and
communication in mental health

Process	Examples and commentary
Referral	Referrals may originate from: Primary care, e.g. practice nurses, health visitors Specialists, e.g. midwifery services Community-based teams, e.g. social services, housing, education, probation General hospitals, e.g. emergency departments, outpatient clinics
Assessment	Mental health assessment may be undertaken by: Primary care mental health workers CMHTs, e.g. CMHNs, psychiatrists, psychologists Crisis teams, multiprofessional assessment aimed at managing current crisis Specialist teams, e.g. mental health liaison team (general hospital), court diversion, drug and alcohol team
Care planning and treatment	Care planning and treatment is based on the identification of what needs to be achieved, the actions and interventions that need to be taken and the criteria against which improvement or deterioration will be measured and may involve: Physical treatments, e.g. psychotropic medication Psychological approaches, e.g. cognitive behavioural therapy (CBT), anxiety management Physical care and health monitoring, e.g. eating and drinking, smoking cessation Ongoing risk assessment and management
Liaison and collaboration	This is underpinned by: Effective communication within and between teams, e.g. unambiguous referral processes, operational standards for communication to referrer and between agencies Identification of named staff to act as a link between services, e.g. link worker acting as a point of contact between the CMHT and community midwifery teams Identification of a named professional undertaking care coordination responsibilities for service users accepted into the mental health service

commissioning, delivery and evaluation of services. The engagement of users with professionals and services has variously been described as 'user involvement', 'user participation', 'user action' and 'the user movement'; whatever term is used, all illustrate the fundamental shift from viewing individuals as passive recipients of care to people who have a meaningful contribution to make to both their own experience of care and how mental health services are organised (The Mental Health Foundation 2003). Table 4.4 summarises the key principles of user and carer involvement.

There are numerous user-centred local and national initiatives, many of which adopt a much broader perspective than simply focusing on service users, becoming involved in local delivery initiatives. For many groups it is impossible to divorce the concept of being a user (or 'survivor') of the mental healthcare system, from the social, political and gender perspectives that influence the experience of using services and receiving mental healthcare. To this end, there has been a 'politicisation' of the service user movement and a number of organisations reflect this growing structural challenge to the way that mental health services are planned, organised and delivered. Examples of such groups include 'Mad Pride' and 'No Force'.

The specific needs of women within mental healthcare have traditionally been poorly addressed, with limited attention paid to issues of gender inequality, relationship and domestic violence and the ability to exercise personal choice when in need of care. Until the publication of the Department of Health's women's mental health strategy (DoH 2003a), there was little policy guidance on the development of gender sensitive services. In one sense, this needs to be seen in the context of the majority of healthcare (and specifically mental healthcare) being planned and delivered from a white, Eurocentric perspective, with many services continuing to be seen as homophobic and non-person centred (Barcan & Glazier 1997). Issues of gender, race, class, ethnic origin, age and sexuality are all likely to be factors that influence both the individual's perception of mental healthcare, such as whether they feel safe to access services in the first place, as well as the way in which care is planned, organised and delivered. Issues connected with gender and sexuality are often poorly handled by professionals and patients may actively choose not to disclose their sexual preferences for fear of reprisals and concern regarding how it may effect their care and treatment (Corrigan & Matthews 2003, Read 2004). Since 2003 there has been a commitment to providing gender-sensitive services,

Table 4.4   Principles of service user and carer involvement

Practice	Underlying value system
Democratic	Structures are established within the organisation, that involve users and carers. These should be democratic, with users themselves deciding who represents them and how they are represented at trust activities
Accountable	User representatives have a responsibility to both inform and consult other service users about their activity
Equitable	As many users and carers as possible should be involved in the organisation's activities. Some client groups, such as those suffering from dementia, are particularly disadvantaged, therefore particular efforts should be made to include them in trust activity. There needs to be an awareness that service user involvement can become concentrated in the hands of a few select individuals, so effort must be made to engage those who do not belong to user and carer organisations or pressure groups
Varied	Acknowledge the need to develop a variety of formats and processes to include user and carer representation – it is important not to simply limit involvement to participation at meetings
Fair allocation of resources	Involvement should not be limited to certain areas, e.g. inner cities, but resources allocated to facilitate the involvement of those not currently engaged, or who live in rural areas
Comprehensive	Accept and work towards user and carer involvement at all levels of the organisation, e.g. service planning, commissioning, delivery and evaluation; staff recruitment, selection and appointment; staff training and professional development. Those involved need to be trained and supported to participate as equals with trust staff
Paid	Payment needs to be made for user and carer time when involved in trust business, not just the payment of expenses

although recent reports suggest that health trusts and professionals have a lot to do in order to meet the expectations outlined in the government's women's mental health strategy (DoH 2003).

There has been limited attention paid by practitioners and researchers into women's views on the provision of mental healthcare during pregnancy and following childbirth (Dowswell et al 2001). Although, as with all aspects of healthcare there has been a growing focus on service user and patient involvement in the planning and organisation of health services, it is not possible to locate any evidence regarding women's views of perinatal mental healthcare.

The impact of mental illness on partners and carers

Up to 1.5 million people in the UK may be involved in caring for a person with a mental health problem (DoH 1999c), and the impact mental ill health has on partners, carers and family members can be significant and may lead to the other person developing mental health-related problems of their own (Krishnasamy et al 2001). For many partners, who may in fact become 'carers', albeit on a temporary basis, the most common difficulty is in accessing the help and support required from statutory services. In relation to pregnancy and childbirth, the woman's partner may have to assume a temporary role as carer, although there are also large numbers of carers, many of whom are parents of younger adults, who assume a permanent and unpaid caring role (Rethink 2004). Partners of women who have given birth may themselves be at risk of developing a mental health problem, specifically depression and physical-related health difficulties (Harvey & McGrath 1988). The most common difficulties that carers encounter are summarised in Box 4.3.

Box 4.3 The most common problems encountered by carers of people with mental health problems

- Difficulties accessing services
- Available services seen as inappropriate
- Lack of continuity of care
- Insufficient access to talking therapies
- Carers feel under-valued and unsupported by mental health services
- Information and confidentiality problems
- Variability in service quality.

(Rethink 2004)

THE ROLE OF NON-PSYCHIATRIC STAFF IN THE PROVISION OF MENTAL HEALTHCARE

The provision of mental healthcare by non-mental health staff presents a number of challenges, with many professionals, particularly nurses, midwives and health visitors viewing mental health issues as the province of the specialist and not of the generalist. Numerous factors may influence and reinforce this view, including:

- Mental health is seen as 'different' and less tangible than physical healthcare
- Healthcare staff describe a lack of training, lack of skill and lack of time as reasons for not addressing mental health issues in physical care settings
- Feelings of professional anxiety and a lack of confidence
- Fear concerning common misapprehensions and stereotypical views of people with mental health problems (The Mental Health Foundation 2000)
- Health and social care practice and educational systems that have been established to care for people with either physical care needs, or mental care needs – militating against the provision of holistic care (Harrison & Hart 2006).

All of the above have the potential to provide a structural barrier to the provision of holistic care and underline the need to look beyond the practice of the individual professional, but at the systems and structures that have the potential to block the ability of healthcare staff to address this need. Having said that, it is also important that all health staff focus on the needs of the individual and how these can be met, as opposed to maintaining rigid professional or service boundaries.

This is particularly important in the provision of effective mental healthcare during the perinatal period, as there is evidence that women and families are often poorly served if they experience a mental health problem during pregnancy and following childbirth. The prevalence of mental health difficulties connected with physical health problems and illnesses is high, with significant rates of depression, anxiety and post-traumatic stress disorder during the perinatal period (Currid 2004). This makes it all the more vital that there are effective arrangements in place to ensure that there is appropriate screening, assessment, treatment and support for mothers and families at this time, although both midwifery and mental health services have been criticised for poor inter-service and cross agency collaboration (Royal College of Psychiatrists 2000).

The NSF for Mental Health (DoH 1999a) requires organisations to develop protocols which address early detection and management of such problems in primary care, through to specialist treatments in maternity units and secondary care services. In order to ensure integrated care from early pregnancy through to the postpartum period, a number of recommendations have been made that focus on early detection of psychiatric morbidity and prompt intervention, alongside coordinated and collaborative care. Regardless of national or local models of care provision, midwives and health visitors maintain a pivotal role in supporting mothers and families during this time. A number of organisations have taken a proactive approach and have developed services that have responded to this public health agenda and service gap. Examples such as those linked to 'Sure Start' programmes and inter-service 'fast track' referral systems demonstrate the development of innovative and creative approaches to meeting perinatal mental health needs (Davies et al 2003). In order to ensure that there is effective inter-service communication, collaboration and liaison, it is important to work within a key values framework that will ensure that the needs of women and families are met during this stage of the life cycle (Box 4.4).

Box 4.4 Values framework underpinning effective inter-service collaboration in relation to perinatal mental healthcare

- A commitment to collaboration and interdisciplinary working between and within healthcare teams, in particular effective liaison and joint working between primary healthcare, secondary mental health and maternity services. Such cross boundary working needs to be supported by appropriate policy and practice guidelines
- Maternity and primary care staff who maintain an up-to-date knowledge and skills base regarding mental health issues, treatment and care
- Development of specialist roles within primary care and maternity teams that focus on mental healthcare
- Willingness by staff to challenge and stretch the boundaries of current professional practice, with the aim of delivering user-led care that meets the needs of women, children and families.

(Blofield 2006)

Despite the problems with the provision of much perinatal mental healthcare, there is a potentially vital role for midwives and health visitors in meeting the needs of women during this period. However, there are a number of issues that these practitioners need to address in order to respond appropriately:

- The need to accept responsibility for contributing to the provision of mental healthcare for their client group
- Ensure appropriate education, professional preparation, clinical supervision and support in order to undertake this aspect of their role
- Develop local 'champions' or specialists within teams and services to act as a resource and support for colleagues and other disciplines
- Develop links with, and maintain networks with mental health professionals on a local basis – consider also the development of care maps or pathways, highlighting the woman's care journey should she be in need of mental health input
- Consider developing skills and knowledge based around the '4-tier' model of intervention (Table 4.5).

The 4-tier model provides a framework for the non-psychiatric professional to consider how they are able to most effectively meet the needs of women with mental health problems during the perinatal period. The four tiers relate to the various levels of knowledge, skill and expertise that the health professional possesses and reinforces the holistic and collaborative approach to mental healthcare during this period, while at the same time, clearly recognising and delineating the responsibilities of mental health practitioners. Level 1 focuses on awareness, recognition and assessment within routine health and maternity care. Within this level, it is essential that every practitioner is able to recognise mental distress and know how to refer on for more specialist advice. All professional groups caring for women during pregnancy and following childbirth should possess these fundamental skills. Level 2 identifies the importance of specific screening and the use of adapted psychological techniques when appropriate. Within level 3 there is an acknowledgment that the professional is working at a specialist or advanced level and following assessment, is able to utilise specific treatment strategies to manage mild to moderate mental health needs. Level 4 is the province of the mental health professional who offers specialist assessment and intervention, working across services and

Table 4.5 Model of practice for meeting mental health needs during pregnancy and following childbirth

Level	Staff group	Assessment activity	Interventions and care
1	All health and social care professionals	Ability to recognise basic mental health need	Effective information giving. Effective communication. Knowing where and how to refer on for specialist assessment (Stillman-Lowe 1997)
2	Health and social care professionals with additional expertise, e.g. midwives	Screening for psychiatric pathology and mental distress	Using adapted psychological techniques such as problem-solving (Read et al 2003)
3	Health professionals with specialist skills, e.g. supervisor of midwives, consultant midwives	Screening and use of specific assessment instruments	Counselling and specific psychological interventions, e.g. anxiety management, problem-solving – delivered within a specific theoretical framework (Bloom 2002)
4	Mental health specialists	Specialist assessment and diagnosis of psychopathology	Specialist psychological support and mental healthcare, e.g. by CMHNs, clinical psychologists, psychiatrists

Self-help and informal support

Adapted from the National Institute for Clinical Excellence 2004 using the skills of consultation and liaison to ensure effective collaborative care.

CONCLUSION

Within this chapter we have seen how mental health services have developed and expanded since early times, and it has identified how lack of care was first replaced by institutional care, and then community-based care. There has been a fundamental shift in the way in which mental distress has been viewed over the centuries, to today's more enlightened and inclusive philosophy of mental healthcare. However, people with mental health problems continue to face discrimination and stigma, as well as experiencing disengagement from society in general and mainstream health and social care in particular. The development of the service user movement since the 1980s has forced health professionals and health policy-makers to address the needs of those who experience mental health problems from the perspective of the individual. Mental health services have continued to develop and grow since 1997, underpinned by a raft of policy and practice guidance, healthcare guidelines and reports and reviews of high-risk groups, such as women during pregnancy and following childbirth.

This chapter has also explored the role of the non-mental health staff in the provision of mental healthcare, underlining the reality that the prevalence of mental distress is so high that all health professionals need to accept that this is a core part of their professional practice. The importance of utilising a collaborative approach to the issue, alongside the development of specific skills is of vital importance if the needs of women during this crucial stage of the life cycle are to be met effectively.

References

Barcan L, Glazier S 1997 User issues and critical theories. In: Tomas B, Hardy S, Cutting P (eds) Mental health nursing: principles and practice. Mosby, London, p 45–56

Blofield A 2006 Perinatal and maternal mental health. In: Harrison A, Hart C (eds) Mental healthcare for nurses: applying mental health skills in the general hospital. Blackwell Publishing, Oxford, p 148–165

Bloom J 2002 Not waving but drowning: mothers in distress. British Journal of Midwifery 10:324–328

Corrigan P, Matthews A 2003 Stigma and disclosure: implications for coming out of the closet. Journal of Mental Health 12:235–248

Currid T J 2004 Improving perinatal mental healthcare. Nursing Standard 19:40–43

Davies B, Howells S, Jenkins M 2003 Early detection and treatment of postnatal depression in primary care. Journal of Advanced Nursing 44:248–255

Department of Health 1999a National service framework for mental health. DoH, London

Department of Health 1999b Saving lives: our healthier nation. DoH, London

Department of Health 1999c Caring about carers: a national strategy for carers. DoH, London

Department of Health 2003a Mainstreaming gender and women's mental health: implementation guidance. DoH, London

Department of Health 2003b Essence of care: patient-focused benchmarks for clinical governance. DoH, London

Department of Health 1990 The care programme approach for people with a mental illness referred to the specialist psychiatrist services. HMSO, London

Department of Health 1998 Modernising mental health services. DoH, London

Department of Health 2000 The NHS plan. DoH, London

Department of Health 2001 National service framework for older people. DoH, London

Department of Health 2002 The national suicide prevention strategy for England. DoH, London

Department of Health 2004 National service framework for children, young people and maternity services. DoH, London

Dowswell T, Renfrew M J, Gregson B et al 2001 A review of the literature on women's views on their maternity care in the community in the UK. Midwifery 17:194–202

Ford R 2004 The policy and service context for mental health nursing. In: Norman I, Ryrie I (eds) The art and science of mental health nursing. Open University Press, Buckingham, p 99–127

Goffman E 1961 Asylums: essays on the social situation of mental patients and other inmates. Penguin, Toronto

Harrison A, Hart C 2006 Mental healthcare for nurses: applying mental health skills in the general hospital. Blackwell Publishing, Oxford

Harvey I, McGrath G 1988 Psychiatric morbidity in spouses of women admitted to a mother and baby unit. British Journal of Psychiatry 152:506–510

Hayes N 2000 Foundations of psychology. Thompson Learning, London

King's Fund 2005 Mental health briefing, 1 March. Online. Available: http://www.kingsfund.org.uk/news/briefings/mentalhealth.html

Krishnasamy M, Wilkie E, Haviland J 2001 Lung cancer healthcare needs assessment. Patients' and informal carers' responses to a national mail questionnaire survey. Palliative Medicine 15:213–227

Ministry of Health 1945 Report of the sub-committee on mental nursing and the nursing of the mentally defective. HMSO, London

National Collaborating Centre for Women's and Children's Health 2003 Antenatal care: routine care for the health pregnant woman. RCOG Press, London

National Institute for Clinical Excellence, The Scottish Executive Health Department and The Department of Health Social Services and Public Safety: Northern Ireland 2004 The confidential enquires into maternal deaths in the United Kingdom. Why mothers die 2000–2002. RCOG Press, London

National Institute for Clinical Excellence 2004 Improving supportive and palliative care for adults with cancer. NICE, London

Nolan P 1993 A history of mental health nursing. Chapman & Hall, London

Norman I, Ryrie I 2004 Mental health nursing: origins and orientations. In: Norman I, Ryrie I (eds) The art and science of mental health nursing. Open University Press, Maidenhead, p 66–98

Onyett S, Smith H 1998 The structure and organisation of community mental health teams. In: Brooker C, Repper J (eds) Serious mental health problems in the community. Ballière Tindall, London, p 62–86

Pilgrim D, Rogers A 1999 A sociology of mental health and illness, 2nd edn. Open University Press, Buckingham

Read J 2004 Sexual problems associated with infertility, pregnancy and ageing. British Medical Journal 329:559–561

Read S, Stewart C, Cartwright P et al 2003 Psychological support for perinatal trauma and loss. British Journal of Midwifery 11:484–488

Rethink 2004 Living with severe mental health and substance use problems. Rethink, Kingston-upon-Thames

Royal College of Psychiatrists 2000 Perinatal mental health services (CR88). RCPsych, London

Stillman-Lowe C 1997 Postnatal mental health: a view from the inside. British Journal of Community Health Nursing 2:173

The Mental Health Foundation 2000 Pull yourself together: A survey of the stigma and discrimination faced by people who experience mental distress. Updates 2, 4. MHF, London

The Mental Health Foundation 2003 User-centred initiatives. Updates 4, 13. MHF, London

Turp M 2001 Psychosomatic health. Palgrave, Basingstoke

Yorkshire Television 1979 Rampton – the secret hospital. ITV, 22 May

Chapter 5

Common mental health disorders

Peter Hadwin

INTRODUCTION

Common mental health problems can include depression, generalised anxiety disorder, panic disorder, post-traumatic stress disorder, phobias, obsessive–compulsive disorder, adjustment disorders (WHO 2004). However, to understand mental disorder or illness means being aware of not only people who have been in contact with services due to a mental health issue, but also the wider population who have experienced transient psychological problems or have managed to cope with a longer-standing problem. A common approach is to use terms such as mild, moderate and severe to describe someone's experience of a mental health problem. However, as Goldberg & Huxley (1992) point out, mild mental health problems can still cause significant distress to the individual. Furthermore, negative terms such as the 'worried well' serve to penalise those who try to cope but may need support to do so. If someone appears to be functioning at a reasonable level and does not display significant levels of distress, then they may be under-assessed for the help and support they need to receive.

Mild to moderate mental health problems are seen as the remit of non-specialist mental health services and are predominantly managed in primary care (SCMH 2005a). Since most maternity care is delivered within the primary care sector, it is essential that midwives and other health workers have some knowledge of the main features of the more common disorders and understand the differentiation between normal pregnancy changes and the anxiety disorders. This chapter will explore some of the common mental health disorders including depression, generalised anxiety disorder, panic disorder, post-traumatic stress disorder, phobias and obsessive–compulsive disorder. Mechanisms for identification of these disorders will be considered along with appropriate care and treatment. However, the focus will be on the idea of holism or the whole person approach (DoH 2003) to mental healthcare, and take the perspective in which the individual's mental health is not thought of as being in a discrete category but as a response specific to the situation she is in.

ANXIETY DISORDERS

Stress and anxiety can have a negative effect on pregnancy, although the precise mechanisms are not clear (Cohen & Nonacs 2005). The effects include placental abruption, premature labour, low Apgar score and low birth weight (Cohen et al 1989, Crandon 1979, Istvan 1986).

Case study: JANE

Jane talks to her friend frequently about feeling concerned and worried about the pregnancy. She fears that the baby may have a problem, as she had drunk large amounts of alcohol around the time of conception. She is having trouble sleeping, is pre-occupied with these thoughts, has a slight tremble, is sweating more than usual and feels constantly jittery about different areas of her life; she is irritable, restless and has poor concentration.

Jane's anxieties and fears are not unusual among pregnant women; modest to moderate levels of anxiety during pregnancy are common (Cohen & Nonacs 2005), as are anxious thoughts and physical symptoms that mimic anxiety such as increased heart rate (Kelly & Little 2001). However, Kelly & Little (2001) differentiate between normal and pathological anxiety. Specific anxious thoughts about the mother and baby are seen as normal but more generalised thoughts of anxiety about other elements of her life are not. This also includes whether the woman feels that this experience is exceeding her coping strategies and whether it is unusual for her to be experiencing such symptoms.

However, there is not a strong evidence base about the effect of pregnancy on mood disorders (Cohen & Nonacs 2005). There is a strong emphasis on researching depression in the perinatal period, but it has been argued that there is a distinct group of patients who present with sub-threshold mixed anxiety and depression (Barlow & Campbell 2000). Therefore, health professionals will need to be more open in the assessment of an individual's experience of their own well-being when pregnant women present with symptoms that do not meet the diagnostic criteria for either depression or anxiety.

Anxiety disorders are broken down into different diagnostic categories (APA 1994):

- Generalised anxiety disorder
- Panic disorder
- Agoraphobia
- Phobias
- Obsessive–compulsive disorder
- Post-traumatic and acute stress disorder.

Generalised anxiety disorder

Generalised anxiety disorder has a prevalence of 3–4% over a 12-month period, although there is higher prevalence in women than in men, with the mean age of onset as 21 years (Fear 2004). The presenting symptoms may be tension related such as headaches, pounding heart and insomnia. Further features include (APA 1994, WHO 2004):

- Autonomic arousal: dizziness, sweating, dry mouth, stomach pains
- Mental tension: undue worry, feeling tense or nervous, poor concentration, negative thinking patterns
- Physical tension: restlessness, headaches, tremors, inability to relax, chest pain or a feeling of constriction
- Irritability
- Sleep disturbance: difficulty staying or falling asleep or restless unsatisfying sleep.

If these features are applied to Jane (see case study above), it becomes apparent that many are present. However, it is important to recognise that many of her concerns about herself and her baby are normal, but that tremors, restlessness and irritability are not (Kelly & Little 2001). What is crucial is identifying the main problems in partnership with women. This will assist in clarifying the sequence of events and determine the priorities for help that may be needed (NICE 2004a).

Heron et al (2004) found that antenatal anxiety occurs frequently, overlaps with depression and increases the likelihood of postnatal depression. Mild anxiety is often associated with the first trimester and reducing that anxiety may have protective, preventive effects for the fetus. Experiencing severe life events in the first trimester can increase the incidence of congenital abnormalities, while maternal anxiety in the third trimester is linked to behavioural and emotional problems in children (Fear 2004).

Health professionals also need to be aware of co-morbidities – such as anxiety and depression or anxiety and substance misuse, which are common. Jane has told her friend about her fears around her alcohol intake, although it seems that she has not shared this with a health worker. A therapeutic relationship will be crucial, with Jane able to discuss these symptoms with her midwife and gain support and help, if that is what she wishes.

Recognition of mixed anxiety and depression is also important since this is thought to be the most frequent form of common mental health problem (Tyrer 2001). The weekly prevalence of mixed anxiety and depression is 92 per 1000 working adults, as opposed to 28 for depression and 47 for anxiety (ONS 2000, cited in SCMH 2005b). WHO (2004) recognise mixed anxiety and depression as a separate entity to depression and anxiety, although Barkow et al (2004) disagree, feeling that it is not a stable entity. Clearly the crucial factor is not the diagnosis per se, but the recognition of symptoms and problems the woman is experiencing.

NICE (2004b) do not recommend any one specific screening tool for anxiety disorders, citing insufficient evidence to do so.

General questions may include:

- Have you noticed yourself feeling more worried or concerned about things in general than usual?
- Have you suddenly felt panicky without a particular reason?
- Have you been feeling more physically tense with a racing heartbeat or a feeling of dread?

If the answer to any of these is positive, NICE recommend the use of a screening instrument such as Beck's Anxiety Inventory (Beck et al 1988), although they recognise the need for further research to validate use in the longer term.

Panic disorder

Panic disorder affects around 1.5–2.5 % of the population, although there is higher prevalence in women than in men (ratio 3–1.5), with the peak period of onset being between 15–24 years (Fear 2004). However, the prevalence of clinically significant anxiety symptoms during pregnancy has not been well studied (Cohen & Nonacs 2005). They feel that the emergence of panic disorder in the puerperium is not simply coincidental, claiming that there is increased risk of panic symptoms in the postpartum period. Cohen et al (1994) also found that there is a significant increase in panic attacks, occurring in 31–63% of women after delivery. However, others feel that the severity of the symptoms is an important factor, with milder, pre-pregnancy panic more likely to remit in pregnancy than more severe forms (March & Yonkers 2001).

Panic attacks may sometimes happen with generalised anxiety disorder but normally the individual would be also experiencing generalised arousal. However, if there are intermittent episodes of panic and the person takes action to prevent these feelings, then this might be seen as panic disorder (NICE 2004b). Symptoms of panic disorder include (NICE 2004b, WHO 2004):

- Intermittent episodes of panic or anxiety
- Taking action to avoid these feelings
- Spontaneous episodes of severe anxiety that start suddenly, rise rapidly and last from minutes to 1 hour
- Palpitations
- Chest pain
- Sense of choking
- Churning stomach
- Dizziness
- Feelings of unreality
- Feeling detached from oneself
- Fearing impending disaster (e.g. death, going mad, heart attack).

The individual fears further attacks and this can lead to both avoiding places where the attacks have occurred and to there being priming, where the fear of the fear becomes a self fulfilling prophecy.

Case study: CAROLE

Carole seems to be coping reasonably well with her pregnancy, but then, in the supermarket, she suddenly feels uncomfortable and hot. She feels hemmed in and starts to experience dizziness and shortness of breath. She then starts to hyperventilate, as she fears that there is something wrong with her and the baby. She rushes out of the supermarket, leaving her shopping behind. Once outside her feelings start to subside, but she is now very concerned that she is going mad.

In Carole's case, she seems to have classic symptoms of a panic attack. Her experience may lead her to avoid either shops or even potentially to go out at all. One of the most debilitating elements of any mental health problem is the effect it has on the person's confidence and view of themselves. Several physical factors may accompany or exacerbate panic disorder (March & Yonkers 2001):

- Hyperthyroidism
- Hyperventilation
- Sleep deprivation
- Caffeine, alcohol, cannabis and even cold preparations
- Chest pain, including mitral valve prolapse.

March & Yonkers (2001) propose that there is considerable variation in symptoms within individuals, with clustering of symptoms, such as cognitive or cardiovascular clusters, and agoraphobia as a complicating factor. They also suggest that women who do not meet the threshold for diagnosis may be equally as affected as those who do. Support for women who experience symptoms is important and may be dealt with by the family. However, different family arrangements may result in this support being absent, which may lead to a worsening of symptoms (Brockington 1996). Midwives may have a crucial role in supporting women with panic disorder, by promoting self-confidence and self-efficacy in being able to cope with the symptoms. This is where self-help material is useful. An affirming approach should be taken, which includes remaining non-judgemental and stressing the normalcy of the experience.

Phobias including agoraphobia

A phobia is an unreasonably strong fear and avoidance of people, places or events (WHO 2004). A phobia may induce a panic attack and can be differentiated from panic disorder by its specificity in that the phobic reaction will be in reaction to a specific place or event. A useful question is to ask: 'Is there anything that you tend to fear or avoid more than usual?' (WHO 2004).

The DSM-IV also discuss various sub-types of phobia (APA 1994):

- Animal (e.g. particular animals or insects)
- Natural environment (e.g. storms, heights)
- Blood-injection-injury (e.g. seeing blood or other invasive medical procedures)
- Situational (e.g. public transport, tunnels)
- Other (e.g. choking, vomiting).

Phobic reactions may also occur in women who have been sexually abused, specifically in relation to circumstances of the abuse itself (Riley 1995). The crucial factor here is not the diagnostic label but the validation of the person's experience. For example, there could be a very real fear that Carole (case study above) may develop agoraphobia, as a coping reaction to dealing with her panic. Other phobias may develop. Social phobia – the incapacitating experiencing of anxiety in social situations or where the woman may be evaluated or judged is more common in women than men (Fear 2004). Rarely, women may also experience a phobic response to their own infant, or a phobia for pregnancy, which may have resulted from the extreme stress of giving birth (Brockington 1996). However, this may not actually be so, with a misattribution of the avoidance reaction to the stress involved, particularly if the events around the birth were traumatic.

NICE (2004b) do not recommend a specific screening instrument for the assessment of phobias, but Wells (1997) recommends the Fear Questionnaire which is a 15-item instrument covering the 15 most common phobias (Marks & Mathews 1979).

Obsessive–compulsive disorder

Obsessive–compulsive disorder (OCD) has a lifetime prevalence of 2.5% with no increased risk for women over men. OCD symptoms are common in other disorders, e.g. depression (Fear 2004). Its features are (WHO 2004):

- Obsessions: frequent, intrusive, recurrent thoughts or images, over which the person has little or no control
- Compulsions: Repetitive rituals performed to reduce anxiety by warding off the dreaded consequences of the obsessions. These commonly concern contamination, checking, ordering, washing, cleaning and magical thinking.

It has been proposed that pregnancy is a well-recognised risk factor in precipitating OCD (Kalra et al 2005), although it has also been argued that the relationship between OCD and pregnancy may be coincidental, given the common nature of both (Altemus 2001). In one study, pregnancy was associated with the onset of OCD in only 13% of women (Williams & Koran 1997).

Case study: APURNA

Apurna became very anxious about her baby. She feared that he was at risk of becoming contaminated by her and others if she did not rigorously wash her hands at least 25 times before touching him. She also became extremely concerned about him being picked up by others and tried to avoid this if at all possible, by telling relatives that he was about to go to sleep or needed feeding. If it were not avoidable, she would wash his clothes, bedding and anything that had come into contact with the other person. Her thoughts became obsessive and she ruminated about what may happen to her son if she did not protect him. However, she tried to hide her problems from her family, as she felt ashamed and fearful that there was something seriously wrong with her.

Often the obsessive thoughts may be of harm coming to the baby (sometimes from the mother herself). Clearly, Apurna is affected in this way and could benefit from support and treatment. However, there is also an echo of normal anxiety and adjustment to parenthood that may occur in women who have had different lifestyles prior to getting pregnant (Altemus 2001). Another common concern of new mothers is the fear of cot death and the concomitant anxiety, which can become obsessive in nature (Brockington 1996). It must be borne in mind that most people frequently experience different elements of OCD such as intrusive thoughts. However, OCD can be highly debilitating and affects both the health of the woman and the baby, as well as affecting relationships within her support network.

To assess the nature of the problem NICE (2005a) recommend the following questions:

- Do you wash or clean a lot?
- Do you check things a lot?
- Is there any thought that keeps bothering you that you would like to get rid of but cannot?
- Do your daily activities take a long time to finish?
- Are you concerned about putting things in a special order or are you very upset by mess?
- Do these problems trouble you?

For women who are pregnant, it is important that midwives recognise and discuss with them whether the behaviours identified above are appropriate or are compulsive, in which they would have little or no control. The experience of OCD in pregnancy is also highlighted in Chapter 1.

Post-traumatic stress disorder

Post-traumatic stress disorder (PTSD) is characterised by the experience of an exceptionally distressing event (brief, prolonged or repeated) that would probably distress anyone who experienced it (WHO 2004). In defining PTSD, there are three key factors that are experienced for at least 1 month:

- Intrusion of thoughts, memories, flashbacks (in which the person seems to re-experience the distressing event) and nightmares
- Avoidance of reminders, similar situations or events, emotional numbness and blunting, detachment from other people
- Increased arousal such as hypervigilance, increased startle, irritability, insomnia and impaired concentration.

Acute stress disorder or reaction is a further derivative: it is more transient, normally not lasting longer than 4 weeks, although the clinical features are very similar (Bowles et al 2000). The risk of developing PTSD is relatively high in women, affecting 20% of those experiencing traumatic events with a lifetime prevalence of 7.8% (Fear 2004). Those with a history of mental health problems are more likely to develop PTSD. There are also other documented risk factors (Ayers 2004):

- Personal and family history of psychopathology
- History of physical and sexual abuse
- Low level of intelligence
- Neuroticism.

Event risk factors:

- Increased dissociation during the event
- Elevated heart rate during the event.

Post-event risk factors:

- Low level of support.

Low levels of the stress hormone cortisol have also been linked to increased susceptibility to PTSD. A study of pregnant women who developed PTSD after 9/11 found that their children had lower than normal levels of cortisol (Yehuda et al 2005). NICE (2005b) recommend that targeted screening in higher risk populations is undertaken. The Trauma Screening Questionnaire (Brewin et al 2002) consists of the ten re-experiencing and arousal items modified to provide only two response options (Box 5.1).

Box 5.1   Trauma screening questionnaire

Please indicate (Yes/No) whether or not you have experienced any of the following at least twice in the past week.
1. Upsetting thoughts or memories about the event that have come into your mind against your will.
2. Upsetting dreams about the event.
3. Acting or feeling as though the event was happening again.
4. Feeling upset by reminders of the event.
5. Bodily reactions (such as fast heartbeat, stomach churning, sweatiness, dizziness) when reminded of the event.
6. Difficulty falling or staying asleep.
7. Irritability or outbursts of anger.
8. Difficulty concentrating.
9. Heightened awareness of potential dangers to yourself and others.
10. Being jumpy or being startled at something unexpected.

(Brewin et al 2002)

There may be a possible link between labour and PTSD (Kelly & Little 2001). The hypothesis is that a difficult or traumatic birth may act as a significant stressor in a fashion similar to known stressors, such as violence or war. Living through this experience might trigger the symptoms of PTSD (i.e. re-experiencing the traumatic event, increased arousal and avoidance of stimuli associated with the event). It is thought that 2–6% of women will experience a PTSD reaction at some point in the early period after childbirth (Cohen et al 2004)). However, Cohen & Nonacs (2005) feel that this area is under-studied and that significant morbidity exists during the postpartum period that may affect future pregnancies. Nevertheless, postpartum stress symptoms appeared to be related more to stressful life events and depression than to pregnancy, labour and delivery (Cohen et al 2004).

Women are vulnerable to PTSD in the pregnancy subsequent to stillbirth, particularly when conception occurs soon after the loss. Turton et al (2001) found that PTSD symptoms were prevalent in the pregnancy that followed a stillbirth. Case level PTSD was associated with depression, state anxiety and conception occurring closer to loss. Symptoms generally resolved naturally by 12 months after the birth of a healthy baby. Subsequent research found a significant relationship between seeing the dead infant and disorganisation of mother-infant attachment in the next-born child at the age of 12 months (Hughes et al 2001). This finding is very relevant since a profound change in clinical practice (seeing and holding the dead infant) has been introduced with great enthusiasm in maternity units in the UK and elsewhere. Turton & Hughes (2002) argue that this was introduced on the basis of limited and non-systematic clinical observation, with the published findings to date not offering any evidence in support of this practice.

DISSOCIATIVE DISORDERS

Dissociative disorders (DD) are a group of psychiatric syndromes characterised by disruptions of aspects of consciousness, identity, memory, motor behaviour, or environmental awareness (Sharon & Sharon 2005). Sidran (2003) describes dissociation as a mental process, which produces a lack of connection in a person's thoughts, memories, feelings, actions, or sense of identity. During the period of time when a person is dissociating, certain information is not associated with other information as it normally would be. DD is linked to either acute or chronic traumatic experiences and thus is closely associated with PTSD. Over 80% of people with DD have a secondary diagnosis of PTSD (Sidran 2003). There are thought to be four types of disorder (APA 1994):

1. Dissociative amnesia characterised by the inability to recall important personal information, usually of a traumatic nature.
2. Dissociative fugue characterised by confusion about personal identity and an inability to recall one's past.
3. Dissociative identity disorder, in which two or more distinct personalities or states are present.
4. Depersonalisation disorder, when the person might feel detached from her own mental processes, as if she is an outside observer of her own body, (although this is experienced by up to 50% of the normal population) (Fear 2004).

A further category may be somatisation disorder, in which physical symptoms are experienced in the absence of physical pathology. Fear (2004) describes the links between the dissociative and somatoform disorders and considers them together. In 1% of the population conversion symptoms can occur when psychological issues are manifested by physical symptoms, including blindness, hallucinations, paralysis or seizures. This is an extremely complex situation and WHO (2004) are careful to advise practitioners to exclude actual physical conditions or depression as a differential diagnosis.

ANTENATAL/POSTNATAL DEPRESSION

When practitioners think of perinatal mental health, postnatal depression (PND) is often the issue they will think of first. Indeed, 15% of postnatal women will experience depression (NICE 2004a). Nicholson (1998) believes that there is no satisfactory explanation as to why PND occurs, working from the assumption that PND is a distinct disorder from depression that affects the general population. However, Fear (2004) mentions there is some debate as to whether PND is really a distinct psychiatric disorder, as it shares many features of depression including (Fear 2004, WHO 2004):

- Tiredness, irritability, anxiety about the baby's welfare
- Tearfulness, low self-esteem
- Feelings of inadequacy and guilt
- Sleep disturbance, lack of appetite
- Thoughts of self harm or suicide

- Vague physical symptoms
- General inability to cope.

There are different approaches to concepts of perinatal mood disorders. WHO (2004) consider that if we try to promote women's mental health by using individual lifestyle risk factors, then we may not address the underlying causes of these factors. This reflects the need to take a holistic view of the person and the system they live in. The alternative is to take an approach of victim blaming, which may increase the very health risks that health workers are trying to reduce, for example, a woman may knowingly take more cocaine to manage the anxiety of being aware of how much harm she was doing to her fetus by taking the cocaine (WHO 2004).

Nevertheless, some awareness of risk factors when applied within a holistic framework can be helpful. Kovalenko et al (2000) defined risk factors as characteristics, variables or hazards that, if present in a person's life, make it more likely that this individual, rather than someone else, will develop a disorder.

Factors for generalised risk for mental ill health are (DoH 2003):

- Poverty
- Employment
- Women's work in the family
- Physical ill health
- Life events
- Social isolation
- Experiences of violence and abuse.

For the perinatal period, Kovalenko et al (2000) further summarised risk factors as enduring psycho-social adversity, a previous history of depression, especially perinatal depression, a lack of an available confidante and an unwanted pregnancy, especially where termination was considered and rejected. However, other factors such as unemployment, lack of support, and physical health problems have been found to be the most important factors associated with a post-partum depressed mood (Rubertsson et al 2005).

Robertson et al (2004) echoed these perceptions, although they revealed a number of methodological and knowledge gaps that need to be addressed in future research. These include examining specific risk factors in women of lower socioeconomic status, risk factors pertaining to teenage mothers.

While the use of risk factors can be helpful, health professionals also need to be mindful of protective factors. Kovalenko et al (2000) defines these as individual and family strengths that protect women and their families from the development of a disorder. Minimal research has so far occurred in this important area, however, potential protective factors for perinatal mood disorders are thought to include (Kovalenko et al 2000):

- Good physical and mental health
- Adequate self-esteem
- An available, supportive interpersonal relationship (especially with partner and with own mother)
- Adequate social and economic circumstances (e.g. housing)
- Transport, access to services, finances and strong community networks
- An uncomplicated delivery, a healthy infant and an infant with an easy temperament.

Case study: KEISHA

In the second trimester, Keisha found that she felt increasingly unable to cope with the physical problems affecting her, in particular her back problems, tiredness and heartburn. Despite discussing these and the negative effects on her mood with her midwife, Keisha did not feel that she was being taken seriously. She felt brushed off and that she was seen to be making a fuss. This seemed to be reinforced by her partner and her family.

After the birth, her incontinence concerned her, as did her back pain. Her thinking became more negative about herself, her ability to care for her baby and her relationship with her partner. Keisha also lost interest in caring for herself and found that her appetite was low. She also gained very little pleasure from anything she did, particularly with her baby. Keisha became more and more uncommunicative and when she did speak to others, she often felt irritable.

For women like Keisha suffering from either antenatal or postnatal depression, the experience of being depressed may bring about feelings of not being a good mother or even failing as a woman. She may have internalised societal perceptions of being able to cope. While it has been important to stress that pregnancy is a normal part of living and not a disease, it has also brought expectations of women that they should be happy, particularly if the baby is seemingly healthy.

An assessment of Keisha's situation, by gathering information to make judgements of which care and treatment are likely to be most effective, should include (Kovalenko et al 2000):

- Physical health
- Personal and family history
- Risk and protective factors
- Current mental state
- Psychological well-being
- Social circumstances and networks
- Relationship issues
- Plans for adjustment to the new life.

Routine screening for postnatal depression has also become popular. The most often used screening tool within perinatal mental health is the Edinburgh Postnatal Depression scale (EPDS) devised by Cox et al (1987). This is used in a variety of different cultures and is widely accepted as a 'gold standard'. There is also the Post Postpartum Depression Screening Scale (PPDS) devised by Tatano and Beck (2001), which is also sensitive and specific. However, the process of screening itself is seen as contentious, with screening tools often used to predict postnatal depression, but not antenatal depression, which has led to a lack of identifying mental health problems in pregnancy (Adams 2004). Furthermore, it is thought that screening tools such as the EPDS and PPDS do not appear to be useful for identifying patients with major or minor depression (Gaynes et al 2004). The National Screening Committee (2005), using evidence from NICE (2003) recommends that the EPDS should not be used as a screening tool during pregnancy. However, it may serve as a checklist as part of a mood assessment for post-natal mothers, when it should only be used alongside professional judgement and a clinical interview.

Questions to ascertain the psychological state of the parents by practitioners might include asking about the following issues (Bennett 2005):

- The level of support available for the woman/parents, their relationship with their extended family and the wider community
- The parents'/mother's feelings about the pregnancy, birth and baby
- How the mother is feeling in herself
- How the father is feeling
- How does the baby seem to be?

BEREAVEMENT

The loss of a child at any developmental stage from embryo to infant and older, can be a traumatic experience. Read et al (2003) feel that healthcare professionals are now becoming more aware of the impact of perinatal death. This awareness is important since Kelly & Little (2001) propose that there is a normal reaction of depression or guilt to miscarriage and that the associated physical symptoms of painful contractions and blood loss are distressing to most women. Bowles et al (2000) found that after spontaneous abortion or miscarriage as many as 10% of women can have acute stress disorder and up to 1% will have post-traumatic stress disorder. However, Parkes (1998) feels that grief at the loss of a pregnancy can become overlooked or ignored.

It may also be important to consider other forms of loss, for example, surrogacy and adoption can also be seen as a form of bereavement. Nicholson (1998) takes the concept even further, suggesting that perceptions of pregnancy and parenthood may include a loss of both occupational and autonomous identity, femininity and sexuality.

WHO (2004) outline how the bereavement process can affect people. They may be preoccupied with the loss, feel overwhelmed by it or present with somatic symptoms. Many of the factors that affect the individual's reaction to the loss are similar to those for other mental health issues:

- The type of loss: this includes fertility issues, miscarriage and termination for varied reasons, including psychological reasons or because of fetal abnormality, stillbirth and neonatal death. The loss may also be related to the effect on the woman's body image, particularly if there is some form of trauma, due to a caesarean or an episiotomy or even if the woman has stretch marks
- The nature of the loss: this includes whether it was unexpected or how much control the woman had over it. If there were concurrent other stresses or other deaths and how traumatic it was, both physically and psychologically
- The individual and the social context: this might include previous experience of loss and the level and availability of family and social support.

Reactions in bereavement are similar to depression. These are low mood; disturbed sleep pattern; loss of appetite; disinterest; withdrawal; feelings of guilt, particularly about actions not taken, which might be seen as preventing the loss; transient hallucinations of the deceased; thoughts of joining the deceased. There might also be an increased use of alcohol or drugs.

APPROACHES TO TREATMENT AND MANAGEMENT OF CARE

Approaches to treatment may be varied according to the nature of the problem. However, Milgrom et al (1999) outline a treatment approach for postnatal depression that may also be applicable to other perinatal mental health problems. Their approach is comprehensive and integrated and outlines three phases:

- Extended assessment
- Goal setting
- Treatment.

The authors stress the importance within the assessment phase of developing rapport with the woman, allowing her time and freedom to tell her story (Milgrom et al 1999). Assessment is the starting point of the therapeutic relationship. The development of the therapeutic relationship is a fundamental and crucial element to mental health. Rogers (1961) believed this was a necessary condition for helping a person to enhance their mental well-being. A therapeutic relationship is about communication and contact but it is also about understanding and clarity. The worker and the individual with a mental health problem need to agree goals and the tasks need to achieve those goals, as well as creating a bond (Bordin 1979). Trust, honesty and openness are also critical elements (Rogers 1961). For women to share their fears and anxieties with midwives or other workers, they will need to feel trust and belief in them. Also necessary is mutual respect of each other's values and beliefs. This is especially important when considering issues of culture, particularly if there is a spiritual belief that may be guiding or influencing women's approaches to their pregnancy.

The key skills required are observation, listening and responding to women's communications: verbal, non-verbal and para-verbal. Active listening skills enable midwives and other workers to make an accurate, comprehensive initial assessment of women's difficulties (Nelson-Jones 2003). It is essential that this be done collaboratively and respectfully. It may be necessary to liaise with other professionals at an early stage to ensure that there is continuity of care and to minimise multiple assessments (NICE 2005b). Care pathways may also be means of clearly stating the process and responsibility of each worker or organisation.

The stepped care model

As recommended by NICE (2004b) the stepped care model is the overarching model of primary care for individuals with mental health issues (Bower & Gilbody 2005, SCMH 2005b). This can be described as a model of healthcare delivery that helps health professionals deliver the least restrictive, but most effective treatment available. The stepped care model recommends the relevant intensity of treatment for the level of distress and impact on functioning of women. The treatment should be monitored systematically and can be changed if proving ineffective (Table 5.1).

Step 1

If women present with mild problems, then watchful waiting for 2 weeks may be appropriate. This step can be performed with both patients who do not wish to have an intervention and patients who the health professional thinks will recover without an intervention (NIMHE 2004). The process for this should be collaborative. It should be explained to women that there will be monitoring of their problems by both themselves and the midwife, and that if they feel that the situation is worsening, then that they should contact the midwife as soon as possible.

Step 2

In step two, it is important to provide information about the particular issue, both about the problem itself and how it might be resolved. This can be done by signposting, assisting women to find an appropriate local or national voluntary organisation (NIMHE 2004), or with the help of self-help guide books. The self-help guides, which can be accessed from several websites, have the advantage of being shorter and contain basic facts and information. Also included may be exercises to help women to apply the knowledge to themselves, useful relevant addresses, and other websites and organisations. They can also be downloaded free of charge or read online. If women do not have access to a computer,

Table 5.1   The stepped care approach

Who is responsible for care?		What do they do?
Acute mental health wards	Risk to life.	Medication and in-patient care.
Mental health specialists	Treatment resistance and frequent recurrences.	Medication and complex psychological interventions.
GP, counsellor, social worker, psychologist, primary care mental health worker	Moderate or severe disorders.	Medication, brief psychological interventions and support groups.
GP, practice nurse, practice counsellor	Mild disorders.	Active review, self help, CBT, exercise, signposting.
Primary care team	Recognition.	Watchful waiting and assessment.

CBT, cognitive behavioural therapy. Adapted from SCMH 2005b.

then midwives may be able to assist in practical ways. If there are literacy problems or if there are cultural or religion dimensions, then these need to be addressed sensitively and early, possibly with the help of others from the appropriate faith, spirituality or culture.

NIMHE (2004) also recommends group psycho-education. This involves a group treatment, providing information and teaching users about the mental health problem and strategies for managing it (e.g. goal planning and relaxation), however these are not therapeutic groups. Exercise may also be helpful (NIMH 2004), perhaps in conjunction with local leisure centres. However, even informal exercise, such as walking, can also be beneficial.

Step 3

Brief psychological interventions and/or medication may be useful, although NIMHE (2004) believe that, in relation to depression, the risk/benefit ratio probably does not warrant prescribing until step 4 (NIMHE 2004). Cognitive behavioural therapy may be useful either as a formal process of exploring difficulties for each mental health problem or by using the basic techniques of problem solving, activity scheduling and thought challenging. Liaison with specialist services may be helpful, often in an advisory capacity.

Medication can be a useful option, either as a sole treatment or in combination with the treatments outlined above. An indication for medication may be the presence of somatic problems, in particular loss of appetite, disturbed sleep, apathy, retardation of thought and poor concentration.

Women with an ongoing mental health problem may be concerned about having taken medication pre-conceptually or during pregnancy, particularly if the pregnancy was unplanned. Remaining on or commencing medication during the perinatal period may also cause anxiety. Midwives will need to carefully and sensitively discuss any concerns the woman may have. It is crucial that information is provided which is clear, jargon free and balanced.

The principal medications that midwives may need to have a working knowledge of, in regard to common mental health problems, are antidepressants and benzodiazepines. Newer antidepressants include selective serum reuptake inhibitors (SSRIs), which include fluoxetine (Prozac). Older antidepressants are the tricyclics (TCAs). Antidepressants do not treat depression alone; some SSRIs can be used to treat panic disorder, mixed anxiety and depression, OCD, PTSD and phobias. Benzodiazepines have been used in the management of anxiety but SIGN (2002) believe that they should be avoided in the first trimester due to the possibility of fetal malformations, including oral cleft.

Fear (2004) recommends that caution should be exercised in prescribing, as most psychotropic drugs cross the placenta. The greatest risk is in the first trimester (between weeks 3 and 11) of congenital abnormalities, a period when many women are not aware of their pregnancy. However, continued use may also be problematic. SIGN (2002) recommends the following principles:

- Establish a clear indication for treatment
- Use the lowest effective dose for the shortest period necessary
- Use drugs which have the best evidence base
- Assess the risk/benefit ratio for mother and baby/fetus.

Postnatally, women who take medication are likely to be discouraged from breast-feeding, although this may be unnecessary. The principles above should be followed in making decisions about medication for a lactating woman. If occurring then breast-feeding should take place immediately before taking medication and avoided 1–2 h after, as plasma concentrations are then at their highest. This can be achieved by taking medication as a single dose before the baby's longest sleep period. It has been suggested that there is no clinical indication to stop breast-feeding when taking either TCAs or SSRIs, provided that the baby is healthy and progress is monitored (SIGN 2002). However, Levinson-Castiel et al (2006) found that one-third of babies whose mothers took antidepressants showed neonatal abstinence syndrome, which has the symptoms of tremors, disturbed sleep and high-pitched crying.

Steps 4 and 5

At these stages, specialist mental health services will normally be involved. This may be in the form of case managers, at step 4 supporting women when at least two evidence-based interventions have not been successful, or in step 5, where women will have been admitted to an inpatient unit, due to a high level of risk and of complex needs, or where the mental health problem has become chronic or treatment resistant.

CONCLUSION

Mental health disorders are common in pregnancy and the postnatal period. For any woman and her baby, it is important she receives support, help and guidance for any psychological issue she is experiencing. The stepped care model outlines how the right level of intervention should be used at the right time for the right problem (SCMH 2005b). This approach can help a woman retain control in a responsive, supportive framework to enhance her ability to cope and resolve her psychological issues. Using evidence-based interventions is challenging, as the evidence is variable and not always clear. However, it is important that the midwife and others involved with the woman's care work with her in an individualistic way, based on her needs, giving her as much informed choice as possible.

References

Adams C 2004 Routine antenatal care for healthy pregnant women. Online. Available: http://www.msfcphva.org/clieffectiveness/cliefniceanteguide.pdf 2 Jan 2006

Altemus M 2001 Obsessive-compulsive disorder during pregnancy and postpartum. In: Yonkers K, Little B (eds) Management of psychiatric disorders in pregnancy. Arnold, London, p 149–163

American Psychiatric Association 1994 Diagnostic criteria from DSM-IV. APA, Washington

Ayers S 2004 Delivery as a traumatic event: prevalence, risk factors, and treatment for postnatal posttraumatic stress disorder. Clinical Obstetrics and Gynecology 47:552–567

Barkow K, Heun R, Wittchen H U et al 2004 Mixed anxiety-depression in a 1 year follow-up study: shift to other diagnoses or remission? Journal of Affective Disorders 79:235–239

Barlow D H, Campbell L A 2000 Mixed-anxiety depression and its implications for models of mood and anxiety disorders. Comprehensive Psychiatry 41(suppl 1):55–60

Beck A T, Epstein N, Brown G et al 1988 An inventory for measuring clinical anxiety: psychometric properties. Journal of Consulting and Clinical Psychology 56:893–897

Bennett R 2005 Guidelines for the identification and management of antenatal and postnatal depression. Online. Available: http://www.bristolnorthpct. nhs.uk/publications/policies_&_procedures/clinical/postnatal_depression/ postnatal%20depression%20guidelines%20april%20'05.d

Bordin E S 1979 The generalisability of the psychoanalytical concept of the working alliance. Psychotherapy Theory Research and Practice 16:252–260

Bower P, Gilbody S 2005 Stepped care in psychological therapies: access, effectiveness and efficiency. British Journal of Psychiatry 186:11–17

Bowles S V, James L C, Solursh D S et al 2000 Acute and post-traumatic stress disorder after spontaneous abortion. American Family Physician 15:1689–1696

Brewin C R, Rose S, Andrews B et al 2002 Brief screening instrument for post-traumatic stress disorder. British Journal of Psychiatry 181:158–162

Brockington I 1996 Motherhood and mental health. Oxford University Press, Oxford

Cohen L S, Nonacs R M (eds) 2005 Mood and anxiety disorders during pregnancy and postpartum. Review of psychiatry, Vol 24, No. 4. American Psychiatric Publishing, Arlington, Virginia

Cohen L S, Rosenbaum J F, Heller V L 1989 Panic attack-associated placental abruption: case report. Journal of Clinical Psychiatry 50:266–267

Cohen L S, Sichel D A, Dimmock J A 1994 Postpartum course in women with pre-existing panic disorder. Journal of Clinical Psychiatry 50: 289–292

Cohen M M, Ansara D, Schei B et al 2004 Posttraumatic stress disorder after pregnancy, labour and delivery. Journal of Women's Health 13:315–324

Cox J L, Holden J M, Sagovsky R 1987 Detection of postnatal depression: development of the Edinburgh postnatal depression scale. British Journal of Psychiatry 150:782–786

Crandon A J 1979 Maternal anxiety and neonatal well being. Journal of Psychosomatic Research 23:113–115

Department of Health 2003 Mainstreaming gender and women's mental health, implementation guide. DoH, London

Fear C 2004 Essential revision notes in psychiatry for MRCPsych. PasTest, Knutsford

Gaynes B N, Gavin N, Meltzer-Brody S et al 2004 Perinatal depression: prevalence, screening accuracy, and screening outcomes. Evidence Report/Technology Assessment Number 119. Online. Available at: http://www.ahrq.gov/clinic/epcsums/peridepsum.pdf 4 Feb 2006

Goldberg D, Huxley P 1992 Common mental disorders. Tavistock/Routledge, London

Heron J, O'Connor T G, Evans J et al; The ALSPAC Study Team 2004 The course of anxiety and depression through pregnancy and the postpartum in a community sample. Journal of Affective Disorders 80:65–73

Hughes P, Turton P, Hopper E et al 2001 Disorganised attachment behaviour among infants born subsequent to stillbirth. Journal of Child Psychology and Psychiatry 42:791–801

Istvan J 1986 Stress, anxiety and birth outcome: a critical review of the evidence. Psychological Bulletin 100:331–348

Kalra H, Tandon R, Trivedi J K et al 2005 Pregnancy-induced obsessive compulsive disorder: a case report. Annals of General Psychiatry 4:12

Kelly M, Little B 2001 Obstetrics for the non-obstetrician. In: Yonkers K, Little B (eds) Management of psychiatric disorders in pregnancy. Arnold, London, p 17–63

Kovalenko N, Barnett B, Fowler C et al 2000 The perinatal period: Early interventions for mental health. In: Kosky R, O'Hanlon A, Martin G, Davis C (eds) Clinical approaches to early intervention in child and adolescent mental health, Vol. 4. Australian Early Intervention Network for Mental Health in Young People, Adelaide

Levinson-Castiel R, Merlob P, Linder N et al 2006 Neonatal abstinence syndrome after in utero exposure to selective serotonin reuptake inhibitors in term infants. Archives of Pediatric and Adolescent Medicine 160:173–176

March D, Yonkers K A 2001 Panic disorder. In: Yonkers K, Little B (eds) Management of psychiatric disorders in pregnancy. Arnold, London, p 134–148

Marks I M, Mathews A M 1979 Brief standard self-rating for phobics. Behaviour Research and Therapy 17:263–267

Milgrom J, Martin P R, Negri L M 1999 Treating postnatal depression. John Wiley, London

NICE 2005a Obsessive compulsive disorder: Core interventions in the treatment of obsessive compulsive disorder and body dysmorphic disorder. Full Guideline. Online. Available: http://www.nice.org.uk/page.aspx?o=289817 12 Dec 2005

NICE 2005b Anxiety: management of post-traumatic stress disorder in adults in primary, secondary and community care. Online. Available: http://www.nice.org.uk/page.aspx?o=CG026fullguideline 10 Jan 2006

NICE 2003 Antenatal care: routine care for the healthy pregnant woman. Online. Available: http://www.nice.org.uk/page.aspx?o=CG006fullguideline 12 Jan 2006

NICE 2004a Antenatal and postnatal mental health: clinical management and service guidance. http://www.nice.org.uk/page.aspx?o=232805 12 Jan 2006

NICE 2004b CG22 Anxiety: full guideline. Online. Available: http://www.nice.org.uk/page.aspx?o=cg022fullguideline 12 Dec 2005

National Institute for Mental Health in England 2004 Enhanced services specification for depression under the new GP contract: a commissioning guidebook. NIMH. Online. Available: http://nimhe.csip.org.uk/index.cfm?fuseaction=main.viewItem&intItemID=28472 10 Jan 2006

National screening committee 2005 Postnatal depression screening. Policy Position – May. National screening committee. Online. Available: http://www.library.nhs.uk/screening/ViewResource.aspx?resID=60978&tabID=288 10 Jan 2006

Nelson-Jones R 2003 Basic counselling skills: a helper's manual UK. SAGE, London

Nicholson P 1998 Post-natal depression: psychology, science and the transition to motherhood. Routledge, London

Parkes C M 1998 Coping with loss: bereavement in adult life. British Medical Journal 316:856–859

Read S, Stewart C, Cartwright P et al 2003 Psychological support for perinatal trauma and loss. British Journal of Midwifery 11:484–488

Riley D 1995 Perinatal mental health. Radcliffe Medical, Oxford

Robertson E, Grace S, Wallington T et al 2004 Antenatal risk factors for postpartum depression: a synthesis of recent literature. General Hospital Psychiatry 26:289–295

Rogers C 1961 On becoming a person: a therapist's view of psychotherapy. Constable, London

Rubertsson C, Wickberg B, Gustavsson P et al 2005 Depressive symptoms in early pregnancy, two months and one year post-partum-prevalence and psychosocial risk factors in a national Swedish Sample. Archive of Women's Mental Health 8:97–104

Sainsbury Centre for Mental Health 2005a The neglected majority: developing intermediate mental health in primary care. SCMH, London

Sainsbury Centre for Mental Health 2005b The neglected majority (policy paper). SCMH, London. Online. Available: http://www.scmh.org.uk/80256FBD004F3555/vWeb/flKHAL6HTLGC/$file/neglected+majority+policy+paper.pdf 10 Jan 2006

Scottish Intercollegiate Guidelines Network 2002 Postnatal depression and psychosis UK. SIGN, Edinburgh

Sharon I, Sharon R 2005 Dissociative disorders. Online. Available: http://www.emedicine.com/med/topic3484.htm 10 Jan 2006

Sidran J 2003 Dissociative disorders. Online. Available: http://www.sidran.org/didbr.html 10 Dec 2005

Tatano C, Beck R 2001 Further validation of the postpartum depression screening scale. Nursing Research 50:155–164

Turton P, Hughes P 2002 Post-traumatic stress disorder and management of stillbirth (correspondence). British Journal of Psychiatry 180:279

Turton P, Hughes P, Evans C D H et al 2001 Incidence, correlates and predictors of post-traumatic stress disorder in the pregnancy after stillbirth. British Journal of Psychiatry 178:556–560

Tyrer P 2001 The case for cothymia: mixed anxiety and depression as a single diagnosis. British Journal of Psychiatry 179:191–193

Wells A 1997 Cognitive therapy of anxiety disorders a practice manual and conceptual guide UK. John Wiley, Chichester

Williams K E, Koran L M 1997 Obsessive-compulsive disorder in pregnancy, the puerperium, and the premenstruum. Journal of Clinical Psychiatry 58:330–336

World Health Organization 2004 WHO guide to mental and neurological health in primary care: a guide to mental and neurological ill health in adults and children and adolescents. UK Royal Society of Medicine Press, London

Yehuda R, Mulherin Engel S, Brand S R et al 2005 Transgenerational effects of posttraumatic stress disorder in babies of mothers exposed to the World Trade Center attacks during pregnancy. Journal of Clinical Endocrinology and Metabolism 90:4115–4118

Chapter 6

Serious mental illness and the midwife

Nigel Philip Weeks

INTRODUCTION

This chapter is concerned with the impact of pregnancy and child-birth on the development or exacerbation of serious mental illness and what midwives can do to help. This requires an understanding of common psychiatric conditions. Defining serious mental illness has always been problematic but for the purposes of this chapter, those serious mental illnesses that will be considered are schizophrenia and related psychoses, the affective disorders and puerperal depression and psychosis. First however, there are a number of issues to address.

Traditionally psychotic experiences were viewed as being qualitatively very different from normal experiences. Early classifications of mental disorders distinguished psychoses and neuroses, with neuroses being seen as extensions of normal emotional responses, while psychoses were seen as completely alien reactions governed by disordered biological activity (Bentall 1990). More recent work (e.g. Bentall 2003) has pointed to the continuum of experience so that people who are not mentally ill may have hallucinatory experiences (Romme et al 1992, Romme & Escher 2000), that delusional beliefs may be similar to strongly held 'normal' beliefs (Hemsley & Garety 1986, Peters et al 1999) and that in everyday conversations people exhibit examples of psychotic speech (Fromkin 1975).

The model used to guide understanding within this chapter is the stress-vulnerability model (Zubin & Spring 1977) which was first proposed to explain schizophrenic breakdown and serves as a useful explanation for the interaction of nature and nurture which determines the development of any psychiatric disorder. This model has two components: stress and vulnerability. The first, stress, is a difficult concept to define without reference to stressors and anxiety. It can be considered as the non-specific response to various stressors that impinge on the organism, which can be both positive and negative and can vary in degree. There are two separate components to stress, the general run of the mill stress of living that can be called ambient stress, for example, commuting to work and running slightly late, taking children shopping for school uniforms, etc. and second, the stress that arises from specific life events, including bereavement, marriage and the birth of a child. The second concept is vulnerability which suggests that the make-up of a person arising from both their genetic complement and the life events that have occurred is influential in their vulnerability to mental illness. For some writers, the vulnerability to a disorder is strongly influenced by genetic make-up (Stevens & Price 1996), while for others it is the interaction between the basic biological temperament which is largely inherited and psychological factors that arise during the developmental period (Dinzeo et al 2004, Eklund et al 2004). From this it follows that some people are extremely vulnerable to psychotic disorders, experiencing psychotic illness in periods of limited stress, while others need a great deal of stress to provoke a breakdown. Once someone has had a severe psychotic experience, they may be more vulnerable to breakdown under stressful experiences for a longer period of time, as they slowly recover.

SCHIZOPHRENIA

Schizophrenia is a serious mental illness that affects around four in 100 000 of the population, appearing to affect men and women equally (Saha et al 2005). However, it generally appears 3–5 years later in women with the age of onset peaking in their 20s (Leung & Chue 2000), coinciding with the main reproductive years. In the UK, psychiatrists are often loathe to utilise a diagnosis of schizophrenia, particularly in the early manifestation of psychotic symptoms, so may utilise terms such as 'first-episode psychosis' or just use the term 'psychosis', partly because of the stigmatising and negative connotations associated with the diagnosis of schizophrenia and partly because the diagnosis is unclear. Although the long-term outcome of schizophrenia is often seen as poor, a recent 25 year follow-up (Harrison et al 2001) found that the majority of sufferers have a favourable outcome with a significant number of early unremitting cases achieving a late-phase recovery. What this means is that however severe the illness appears to be, there is a need to retain a therapeutic optimism, for a diagnosis of schizophrenia does not necessarily mean a severe, long-term and unremitting illness.

The symptoms of schizophrenia can be broadly grouped into two clusters: positive and negative (Fenton & McGlashan 1991, Liddle 1987). Positive symptoms are those that are present in people with schizophrenia, such as hallucinations, delusions and thought disorders, while negative symptoms are those symptoms that are absent such as apathy, anhedonia (loss of pleasure) and poverty of speech (the amount of speech that is produced is reduced). It is important to remember that there is no value judgement on the choice of the words 'positive' and 'negative' to describe these symptoms, rather they describe whether or not the features are present or absent. In terms of disability, negative symptoms can often be the most disabling and those that carers find particularly frustrating (Tucker et al 1998), particularly as it can appear that people are being lazy and not trying. It seems likely that the negative symptoms are part of the psychological coping mechanism to deal with the impact positive symptoms may be having, a sort of emotional shut down.

AFFECTIVE DISORDERS

The affective disorders considered in this chapter are the more severe end of the mood disorder spectrum. The American diagnostic system DSM-IV-TR (American Psychiatric Association, APA 2000) which is commonly used refers to three major types of affective disorder: bipolar I, bipolar II and major depressive disorder. Bipolar I is the classical 'manic-depressive psychosis', which consists of recurrent episodes of both depression and mania; bipolar II consists of recurrent episodes of depression with at least one episode of hypomania; and major depressive disorder in which there has never been a hypomanic episode.

The symptoms of severe depression include slowing down of bodily function, which if not treated can lead to stupor, depressed mood for most of the day, loss of interest, loss of appetite and weight, although paradoxically there may be an increase in appetite and weight gain, sleep disturbances, particularly early morning wakening, fatigue or loss of energy, abnormal self reproach or excessive guilt feelings, poor concentration and morbid thoughts.

There may be delusions of guilt, nihilistic delusions (the belief that part of the self does not exist, that the body is empty) and suicide is a real risk (APA 2000).

The symptoms of mania are a persistent and abnormally elevated mood and are the opposite of a depressed mood. There may be increased sense of self worth and ability that is often delusional in nature, there is a reduction in the need for sleep, an increase in activity, the speech is rapid and as if under extreme pressure. Ideas may be linked by puns, similes and other word plays ('flight of ideas') with extreme distractibility; there is an increase in risk-taking and excessive involvement in pleasurable activities. People can become extremely promiscuous, experiment with different drugs and generally demonstrate extremely disinhibited behaviour, for example, they may spend sums of money they do not have or do things that are totally out of character. The behaviour is such that it causes a severe impairment in the person's ability to function normally. There is a real risk of exhaustion if untreated (APA 2000).

Hypomania is similar to mania but is not so severe. The features are of a degree that is noticeably different from the norm but does not cause a severe impairment in a person's ability to function. People's hypomanic symptoms rarely lead them to treatment, while the major distinction with mania is duration (APA 2000). Because of the disinhibition associated with mania and hypomania, women are vulnerable to exploitation. They may engage in relationships that they would not normally do and thus as a consequence there may be increased risk of unwanted pregnancy, of breakdown in stable and supportive relationships and an increase in sexually transmitted disease. In general, women who have a serious mental illness have had more sexual partners, are more likely to have been coerced into unwanted sexual activity including rape, are more at risk for sexual transmitted diseases and are more likely to have had an induced abortion than the general population (Coverdale et al 1997, Raja & Azzoni 2003).

PREGNANCY AND SERIOUS MENTAL ILLNESS

It is important to consider the impact of pregnancy and birth on the development of serious mental illness in more detail. Traditionally mood changes during pregnancy are divided into three groups: the baby blues, postnatal depression and puerperal psychosis (Heron et al 2005). It is debatable whether there is such an entity as puerperal psychosis that is separate from other psychiatric disorders and only associated with pregnancy and birth, or whether pregnancy and birth is such a stressful period that it can lead to the onset of psychosis in vulnerable women. For example, DSM-IV-TR (APA 2000) does not include a category for puerperal psychosis but subsumes it into other diagnostic categories. For DSM-IV-TR (APA 2000), a psychotic disorder must occur within the first month after birth to qualify for postpartum onset. The International Classification of Diseases (ICD-10) (World Health Organization 1992) defines puerperal disorders as those that occur within 6 weeks of birth that cannot be classified elsewhere. The result of this is that it is unclear whether there is a specific severe mental illness that is solely associated with pregnancy.

There is evidence of an association between psychosis and pregnancy. The relative risk of a woman being admitted with a postnatal psychotic illness in the month after birth is approximately 22 times the risk of a women being admitted in the 2 years previous to pregnancy. In addition, with a second birth, that risk increases to 35 times (Kendell et al 1987). In 1–2 per 1000 births, the mother develops a psychosis that requires hospital admission (Kumar et al 1995, Videbech & Gouliaev 1995), although the overall incidence could be in the region of four in 1000 births. Studies seem to suggest that the overwhelming majority of people who are diagnosed with a puerperal psychosis have a bipolar disorder (Brockington et al 1981, Hunt & Silverstone 1995, Jones & Craddock 2001, Videbech & Gouliaev 1995). In a comprehensive review of common mood disturbances in the puerperium, Henshaw (2003) found that weeping was common, with up to 80% of mothers being tearful, which was not necessarily associated with depressed mood. In addition, emotional lability is found with new mothers experiencing frequent mood changes during the day. Confusion and cognitive impairments were also frequently found. Elation in the first couple of days after birth is common with up to 30% of new mothers feeling elated (Heron et al 2005). It is difficult to determine the extent to which this is the happiness of the birth of a new child or indications of a later puerperal affective disorder. Mild hypomania in the immediate postnatal period may be predictive of future puerperal psychosis, although there is a paucity of evidence around the 'highs' associated with childbirth (Heron et al 2005). It is therefore likely that childbirth may be a trigger for the development of bipolar disorder in susceptible women.

For women with existing bipolar disorder, the risk of puerperal psychosis is extremely high, following between 25 and 50% of deliveries in these women, which represents a major increase on that expected (Jones & Craddock 2005).

APPROACHES TO CARE

The care required for people who have a history of serious mental illness must be considered. Women with psychosis have a lower fertility rate than controls, particularly those with a history of schizophrenia (Howard 2005), which may be partly due to women with schizophrenia having less stable relationships and partly the contraceptive nature of antipsychotic medication. However, the majority of women with psychosis are mothers (McGrath et al 1999). Newer antipsychotic medications may have a reduced contraceptive effect (Dickson et al 2000) and together with improved psychosocial treatments, the quality of life for people with psychosis has improved. Thus, the consideration of having a family for women with schizophrenia is a much more real possibility (Allison 2004). There are a number of issues that need to be addressed. They are: the management of medication during pregnancy; the engagement and involvement of potential mothers in their antenatal care; the early detection and management of psychotic symptoms that might arise; the development of bonding with the newborn; and continuing support postpartum.

Potential mothers who have a history of serious mental illness are likely to be in contact with mental health services and have a key-worker who oversees their care plan. This may include regular medication together with other psychosocial interventions such as symptom management, family work and relapse prevention (DoH 1999, NICE 2002). Medication in particular is likely to be a major concern for prospective mothers. They may seek advice from their midwife or their key-worker, so it is important to have an understanding of the issues involved.

Medication

Medication management (Gray et al 2004) is a term that describes the interventions used to help people remain concordant with their prescription regime. There are two main groups of medication that are used in people with psychosis: the neuroleptics and mood stabilisers. People with a history of depression may also be receiving long-term antidepressant medication. Current National

Institute for Clinical Excellence Guidelines (NICE 2002) recommend that for newly diagnosed schizophrenia, the first choices of medication are oral atypical antipsychotics such as risperidone, olanzapine, amisulpride, quetiapine and zotepine. As new mothers are generally in the younger age group these are the medications they are likely to be prescribed. The advice is to avoid these in pregnancy unless the benefits of use outweigh the risks, however the potential for relapse in psychosis if the medication is stopped is quite high. This leads to a dilemma in the sort of advice to give – should the mother-to-be stop taking her medication and risk psychosis, or continue taking the medication and risk fetal damage. Generally speaking, antipsychotic medication should not be suddenly discontinued. The British National Formulary (Mehta 2005) recommends gradually withdrawing the medication under close supervision to prevent acute withdrawal and rebound psychosis, so the advice given may relate to whether or not the pregnancy is planned.

Where pregnancy is planned, it may be possible to plan the reduction in medication over a suitable timescale in order to monitor whether or not psychotic symptoms are arising. However, this is not possible in unplanned pregnancy. In this case, there is the need for careful discussions between the mother, the psychiatric care team and the midwifery team. If antipsychotic medication is suddenly stopped, an acute psychosis may develop leading to hospitalisation, requiring an increased dose of antipsychotic medication. The risk of congenital malformation as a result of continued use of antipsychotic medication is unclear (Allison 2004), with few longitudinal studies having been undertaken.

It has been suggested (Allison 2004) that traditionally, where there is a conflict between the health of the mother and the health of the baby, the mother should make the sacrifice to ensure a healthy child. However, this paternalistic view has been criticised by feminist thinkers. The modern notion of collaborative working central both to the provision of quality psychiatric care and to midwifery services would suggest that a careful individual process needs to take place, that supports the mother in making what may be an invidious decision. The impact of psychosis on people has given rise to post-traumatic stress reactions (Kennedy et al 2002, Stampfer 1990) which may accentuate the fear of relapse, so if the mother decides to take the risk of fetal damage, she must be supported in that decision. The role of the worker therefore is to help the mother and her family weigh up the pros and cons of both continuing antipsychotic medication or discontinuing it, taking into account their perception of the impact of psychosis.

As mood-stabilising drugs have an increased profile in terms of teratogenic effects (Freeman & Gelenberg 2005, Iqbal et al 2001, Viguera et al 2002) so different considerations may apply, although it still must be a carefully considered individual decision. Mood-stabilising drugs commonly used are lithium, sodium valproate and carbamazepine. It may be that pregnancy itself protects some-what from the development of bipolar disorder during pregnancy (Grof et al 2000), although the risk increases markedly after birth, so that reduction in mood-stabilising medication during pregnancy is a possibility. Lithium has been associated with cardiac malfor-mations, in particular the Ebstein anomaly, with the risk being 10–20 times that of the general population (De Santis et al 2004, Kohen 2004). Continued use during pregnancy should be carried out cautiously. Both carbamazepine and sodium valproate have been associated with increased risk of spina bifida of between 1% and 5%, while valproate has also been associated with increased excitability in the newborn (Freeman & Gelenberg 2005, Kohen 2004). The benefits of continuing use therefore, must be weighed against the risks of switching to a less toxic medication or discon-tinuing the prescription altogether. This may also relate to whether the pregnancy was planned or unplanned, but in general it is not advisable to suddenly discontinue such medication.

Dealing with breast-feeding issues is also important, particularly with the drive by professionals to encourage breast-feeding (e.g. Ingram & Johnson 2004, Raine 2003) as a desirable outcome for new mothers. Some will want to breast-feed yet feel uncomfortable about breast-feeding and taking medication. For those who are receiving psychotropic medication breast-feeding may not be desir-able and this again has the potential for conflict. Lithium in partic-ular is expressed in breast milk and is toxic to infants having been associated with changes in electrocardiogram readings, lethargy, cyanosis and hypotonia (Curtis 2005, Worsley 2000), therefore a careful risk-benefit analysis needs to occur. When mothers are depressed and experiencing feelings of guilt, this may be enhanced by the guilt of not being able to breast-feed. A recent study found that there was also an association between finding breast-feeding difficult and postnatal depression, and that interactions between the new mother and professionals were unhelpful and highly charged (Shakespeare et al 2004). Care needs to be taken that the decisions the mother makes related to choice of feeding method are supported.

Engagement

Many people who have had a history of serious mental illness have problems engaging with services for a number of reasons. They may find it difficult to form relationships with people in general, finding meeting new people extremely anxiety provoking. They may have been admitted to hospital under a section of the Mental Health Act and thus find authority very threatening. They may be fearful that having a label of mental illness means that authorities will not let them keep their child. There is evidence to suggest that women with serious mental illness are more likely to have given their children up for care by others (Coverdale et al 1997). These aspects are likely to make them avoid services. Therefore, the midwife needs to be extremely sensitive to the individual needs of each woman. The core conditions underpinning any therapeutic engagement are those of empathy, warmth, genuine and unconditional acceptance, since the better the therapeutic alliance, the better the outcome. Although in most interpersonal relationships the Mnemonic SOLER (Egan 1998) (Sit squarely, Open position, Lean forward, Eye contact, Relax) is thought to encourage effective interactions, people who are suffering schizophrenia in particular may find those sorts of interactions anxiety provoking (Nelson 2005). It might be more appropriate to sit alongside the mother and initially engage with very practical issues. For someone who is suffering from florid psychotic symptoms such as hallucinations and delusions, there may be real problems in concentrating and processing information. It is important therefore for the midwife to recognise this. Recognising that someone has difficulty in processing information means that it may need to be chunked into easily digestible pieces, with a longer time than usual for information digestion (Nelson 2005).

There is a great deal of research (Bebbington & Kuipers 1995, Butzlaff & Hooley 1998, de Jesus Mari & Streiner 1994, Leff et al 2003) that high expressed emotion (HEE) contributes to relapse. The concept of HEE emerged from the work related to understanding why people with schizophrenia who were discharged to their families faired worse than people who were discharged elsewhere (Brown 1985). The emotional climate of the family was explored and a structured interview (known as The Camberwell Family

Interview) was developed. This identified five dimensions that appeared to be important. These dimensions were (Brown et al 1972, Vaughn & Leff 1976):

- Critical comments (CC): A count of the number of critical comments made about the patient during the interview
- Hostility: a measure of the degree of hostility expressed during the interview on a four-point scale, 0–3
- Emotional over-involvement (EOI): A six-point scale, 0–5, that measured the degree of emotional self sacrificing behaviour
- Warmth: also a six-point scale
- Positive remarks: the number of positive comments about the patient made during the interview.

In practice, it is only the first three – CC, hostility and EOI that are significant. Families who rated 6 or more on CC; 1 or more on hostility; and/or 3 or more on EOI are rated as HEE, others as low expressed emotion. It is important to note that these are measures of the families coping style and are not causal in relation to psychosis but rather a maladaptive way of coping with the stress of caring that in fact increases the emotional stress within the family.

There is also more recently, emerging work that the impact of HEE workers is also detrimental, that is workers who respond to the stress of caring for someone who is behaving in a difficult manner by hostile or critical comments (Kuipers & Moore 1995, Tattan & Tarrier 2000, Van Humbeeck et al 2001). It is therefore important to respond in a low expressed emotion way that recognises the illness as genuine and that the symptoms are real for the person and are not in their control. Negative symptoms are particularly difficult, as carers often perceive the person as being lazy and not trying, rather than being disabled by particularly difficult symptoms. Mothers who do not appear to be interested in their newborn child may in fact be quite disabled by a psychiatric disorder, for example, the mother who is experiencing psychotic symptoms that affect the way she interacts with her newborn infant may neglect the child and not respond to its cries.

Low expressed emotion responses would focus on the needs of the mother, by remaining calm and objective and by being non-intrusive and non-confrontational (Vaughn & Leff 1981) Conversely, HEE responses tend to blame the person for their illness using terms such as lazy and uncaring, with the HEE worker often being inflexible in their responses. The midwife therefore must remain calm, warm and engaging, and recognise that these symptoms are because of the altered perception the mother is experiencing.

Risk management

When working with new mothers who have a serious mental illness, a careful risk assessment needs to be undertaken. Although suicide during pregnancy and the postpartum period is less common than in the general female population, there is a much greater risk among women who have been hospitalised with a postpartum psychosis (Lindahl et al 2005, Marzuk et al 1997). Suicide has been identified as a major cause of death among new mothers (NICE 2004, Oates 2003a,b, Sullivan et al 2003). Expressed suicidal thoughts should never be down-played. Talking with people about their suicidal feelings will not make those feelings worse. It is often the case that talking through feelings of suicide in a warm and empathetic way may lesson the feelings of isolation and guilt that contribute to suicide. Routine screening of new mothers with the Edinburgh Postnatal Depression Scale (Cox et al 1987) has been shown to be valuable in detecting depression, following which interventions can be implemented (Davies et al 2003).

While filicide (the killing of a child by a parent) is uncommon it does present as a real risk among new mothers who have a psychiatric disorder. About 10 cases a year occur in the UK (Oates 2003a) in addition to a small number who also commit suicide. Some of these women could be classed as altruistic because they care deeply for their child (Stanton et al 2000). The filicide occurs in the context of disordered thinking with the child seen as being 'better off', and is strongly associated with suicide. It is therefore important to recognise this small risk and it should be borne in mind when assessing postnatal women.

Early intervention

Early detection of psychotic experiences appears to be beneficial in reducing the impact of psychosis on the individual. Therefore, the midwife needs to be alert to identifying such indications. For patients who have had previous mental illness, there may be specific indications that can be termed their relapse signature, which are the warning signs that predict relapse (Nelson 2005). For mothers who have never had a previous episode, the symptoms can vary but usually relate either to mania or to severe depression

(Brockington 2004), and delusional beliefs related to the infant often occur. Careful assessment of risks to the mother and baby needs to be carried out.

There is ample evidence that depression and psychosis has a negative impact on child development (Beck 1998, Burke 2003, Murray & Cooper 1997). Beck (1996) found that depressed mothers erect an emotional barrier between themselves and their infants, and thus do not respond to cues the infants give out. However, a Swedish study (Edhborg et al 2003) found that fathers' interactions with their child compensated for this somewhat. Hipwell et al (2005) found that for 5 year olds, where the mother had postnatal depression, there occurred parental conflict and increased aggressive play behaviour among boys. These studies point to the need for early identification and intervention to try and mitigate these longer-term effects on the child and the family.

Treatment

Modern psychiatric care can be effective in the treatment of perinatal mental illness. A combination of medication and psychotherapeutic approaches, in particular cognitive-behavioural interventions, is effective in the treatment of severe postnatal depression (Gjerdingen 2003). Attempts at preventative interventions have been less successful (Lumley & Austin 2001). Debriefing interventions immediately after birth appear to be ineffective in reducing levels of depression experienced later (Gamble et al 2002), although following the identification of people with non-psychotic depression, some counselling approaches may reduce depression (Holden et al 1989).

CONCLUSIONS

The perinatal period is a time of greatly increased risk for psychiatric disorder, which should not be overlooked. Treatment can be effective once affected women are identified. For generalists and midwives it is important to be able to recognise early indications of mental ill health, and to interact in a warm and genuine manner with the new mother and her family. Central to this approach is the recognition that when a new mother is experiencing severe mental illness it is a frightening experience for all involved. The health professional should adopt a careful and sensitive approach to engagement with the woman and promote a carefully coordinated effort between specialist mental health services and the maternity services.

References

Allison S K 2004 Psychotropic medication in pregnancy: ethical aspects and clinical management. Journal of Perinatal and Neonatal Nursing 18:194–205, 288–291

American Psychiatric Association (APA) 2000 Diagnostic and statistical manual of mental disorders, 4th edn. APA, Washington DC

Bebbington P E, Kuipers E 1995 Predicting relapse in schizophrenia: Gender and expressed emotion. International Journal of Mental Health 24:7–22

Beck C 1996 Postpartum depressed mothers' experiences interacting with their children. Nursing Research 45:98–104

Beck C 1998 The effects of postpartum depression on child development: a meta-analysis. Archives of Psychiatric Nursing 12:12–20

Bentall R 2003 Madness explained: psychosis and human nature. Penguin, London

Bentall R P 1990 Reconstructing schizophrenia. Routledge, London

Brockington I 2004 Postpartum psychiatric disorders. Lancet 363:303–310

Brockington I F, Cernik K F, Schofield E M et al 1981 Puerperal psychosis. Phenomena and diagnosis. Archives of General Psychiatry 38:829–833

Brown G, Birley J, Wing J K 1972 Influence of family life on the course of schizophrenic disorders: a replication. British Journal of Psychiatry 121:241–258

Brown G W 1985 The discovery of expressed emotion: induction or deduction. In: Leff J, Vaughn C (eds) Expressed emotion in families. Guilford Press, New York, p 7–25

Burke L 2003 The impact of maternal depression on familial relationships. International Review of Psychiatry 15:243–255

Butzlaff R L, Hooley J M 1998 Expressed emotion and psychiatric relapse. Archives of General Psychiatry 55:547–552

Coverdale J H, Turbott S H, Roberts H 1997 Family planning needs and STD risk behaviours of female psychiatric out-patients. British Journal of Psychiatry 171:69–72

Cox J L, Holden J M, Sagovsky R 1987 Detection of postnatal depression: Development of the 10-item Edinburgh Postnatal Depression Scale. British Journal of Psychiatry 150:782–786

Curtis V 2005 Women are not the same as men: specific clinical issues for female patients with bipolar disorder. Bipolar Disorders 7:16–24

Davies B R, Howells S, Jenkins M 2003 Early detection and treatment of postnatal depression in primary care. Journal of Advanced Nursing 44:248–255

de Jesus Mari J, Streiner D L 1994 An overview of family interventions and relapse on schizophrenia: Meta-analysis of research findings. Psychological Medicine 24:565–578

De Santis M, Straface G, Carducci B et al 2004 Risk of drug-induced congenital defects. European Journal of Obstetrics Gynecology and Reproductive Biology 117:10–19

Department of Health 1999 National service framework for mental health: modern standards and service models. DoH, London

Dickson R, Seeman M, Corenblum B 2000 Hormonal side effects in women: Typical versus atypical anti-psychotic treatment. Journal of Clinical Psychiatry 61:10–15

Dinzeo T J, Cohen A S, Nienow T M et al 2004 Stress and arousability in schizophrenia. Schizophrenia Research 71:127–135

Edhborg M, Lundh W, Seimyr L 2003 The parent-child relationship in the context of maternal depressive mood. Archives of Women's Mental Health 6:211–216

Egan G 1998 The skilled helper: a problem-management approach to helping, 6th edn. Brooks/Cole, Albany

Eklund M, Hansson L, BengtssonTops A 2004 The influence of temperament and character on functioning and aspects of psychological health among people with schizophrenia. European Psychiatry 19:34–41

Fenton W S, McGlashan T H 1991 Natural history of schizophrenia subtypes. II. Positive and negative symptoms and long-term course. Archives of General Psychiatry 48:978–986

Freeman M P, Gelenberg A J 2005 Bipolar disorder in women: reproductive events and treatment considerations. Acta Psychiatrica Scandinavica 112:88–96

Fromkin V A 1975 'A linguist looks at' schizophrenic language. Brain and Language 2:498–593

Gamble J A, Creedy D K, Webster J et al 2002 A review of the literature on debriefing or non-directive counselling to prevent postpartum emotional distress. Midwifery 18:72–79

Gjerdingen D 2003 The effectiveness of various postpartum depression treatments and the impact of antidepressant drugs on nursing infants. Journal of the American Board of Family Practice 16:372–382

Gray R, Wykes T, Edmonds M et al 2004 Effect of a medication management training package for nurses on clinical outcomes for patients with schizophrenia: cluster randomised controlled trial. British Journal of Psychiatry 185:157–162

Grof P, Robbins W, Alda M et al 2000 Protective effect of pregnancy in women with lithium-responsive bipolar disorder. Journal of Affective Disorders 61:31–39

Harrison G, Hopper K, Craig T et al 2001 Recovery from psychotic illness: A 15- and 25-year international follow-up study. British Journal of Psychiatry 178:506–517

Hemsley D R, Garety P A 1986 The formation of maintenance of delusions: a Bayesian analysis. British Journal of Psychiatry 149:51–56

Henshaw C 2003 Mood disturbance in the early puerperium: a review. Archives of Women 's Mental Health 6(suppl 2):33–42

Heron J, Craddock N, Jones I 2005 Postnatal euphoria: are 'the highs' an indicator of bipolarity? Bipolar disorders 7:103–110

Hipwell H E, Murray L, Ducournau P et al 2005 The effects of maternal depression and parental conflict on children's peer play. Child: Care, Health & Development 31:11–23

Holden J M, Sagovsky R, Cox J L 1989 Counselling in a general practice setting: controlled study of health visitor intervention in treatment of postnatal depression. British Medical Journal 298:223–226

Howard L M 2005 Fertility and pregnancy in women with psychotic disorders. European Journal of Obstetrics, Gynecology, and Reproductive Biology 119:3–10

Hunt N, Silverstone T 1995 Does puerperal illness distinguish a subgroup of bipolar patients? Journal of Affective Disorders 34:101–107

Ingram J, Johnson D 2004 A feasibility study of an intervention to enhance family support for breast feeding in a deprived area in Bristol, UK. Midwifery 20:367–379

Iqbal M M, Sohhan T, Mahmud S Z 2001 The effects of lithium, valproic acid, and carbamazepine during pregnancy and lactation. Journal of Toxicology Clinical Toxicology 39:381–392

Jones I, Craddock N 2001 Familiality of the puerperal trigger in bipolar disorder: results of a family study. American Journal of Psychiatry 158:913–917

Jones I, Craddock N 2005 Bipolar disorder and childbirth: The importance of recognising risk. British Journal of Psychiatry 186:453–454

Kendell R E, Chalmers J C, Platz C 1987 Epidemiology of puerperal psychoses. British Journal of Psychiatry 150:662–673

Kennedy B L, Dhaliwal N, Pedley L et al 2002 Post-traumatic stress disorder in subjects with schizophrenia and bipolar disorder. Journal of the Kentucky Medical Association 100:395–399

Kohen D 2004 Psychotropic medication in pregnancy. Advances in Psychiatric Treatment 10:59–66

Kuipers E, Moore E 1995 Expressed emotion and staff-client relationships: Implications for community care of the severely mentally ill. International Journal of Mental Health 24:13–26

Kumar R, Marks M, Platz C et al 1995 Clinical survey of a psychiatric mother and baby unit: characteristics of 100 consecutive admissions. Journal of Affective Disorders 33:11–22

Leff J, Alexander B, Asen E et al 2003 Modes of action of family interventions in depression and schizophrenia: the same or different? Journal of Family Therapy 25:357–370

Leung A, Chue P 2000 Sex differences in schizophrenia, a review of the literature. Acta Psychiatrica Scandinavica 401:3–38

Liddle P F 1987 The symptoms of chronic schizophrenia. A re-examination of the positive-negative dichotomy. British Journal of Psychiatry 151:145–151

Lindahl V, Pearson J L, Colpe L 2005 Prevalence of suicidality during pregnancy and the postpartum. Archives of Women 's Mental Health 8:77–87

Lumley J, Austin M P 2001 What interventions may reduce postpartum depression. Current Opinion in Obstetrics Gynecology 13:605–611

Marzuk P M, Tardiff K, Leon A C et al 1997 Lower risk of suicide during pregnancy. American Journal of Psychiatry 154:122–123

McGrath J J, Hearle J, Jenner L et al 1999 The fertility and fecundity of patients with psychoses. Acta Psychiatrica Scandinavica 99:441–446

Mehta D K (ed.) 2005 British National Formulary 50, September. Pharmaceutical Press, London

Murray L, Cooper P 1997 Effects of postnatal depression on infant development. Archives Disease in Childhood 77:99–101

National Institute for Clinical Excellence 2002 Schizophrenia: core interventions in the treatment and management of schizophrenia in primary and secondary care. NICE guideline. NICE London

National Institute for Clinical Excellence 2004 Confidential enquiry into maternal and child health, why mothers die 2000–2002. The sixth report of the confidential enquiries into maternal deaths in the United Kingdom. NICE. RCOG Press, London

Nelson H 2005 Cognitive-behavioural therapy with delusions and hallucinations: A practice manual, 2nd edn. Nelson Thorns, Cheltenham

Oates M 2003a Perinatal psychiatric disorders: a leading cause of maternal morbidity and mortality. British Medical Bulletin 67:219–229

Oates M 2003b Suicide: the leading cause of maternal death. British Journal of Psychiatry 183:279–281

Peters E, Day S, McKenna J et al 1999 Delusional ideation in religious and psychotic populations. British Journal of Clinical Psychology 38:83–96

Raine P 2003 Promoting breast-feeding in a deprived area: the influence of a peer support initiative. Health Social Care in the Community 11:463–469

Raja M, Azzoni A 2003 Sexual behaviour and sexual problems among patients with severe chronic psychoses. European Psychiatry. Journal of the Association of European Psychiatrists 18:70–76

Romme M A, Honig A, Noorthoorn E O et al 1992 Coping with hearing voices: An emancipatory approach. British Journal of Psychiatry 161:99–103

Romme R, Escher S 2000 Making sense of voices; A guide for mental health professionals working with voice-hearers. Mind Publications, London

Saha S, Chant D, Welham J et al 2005 A systematic review of the prevalence of schizophrenia. Plos Medicine 2:413–433

Shakespeare J, Blake F, Garcia J 2004 Breast-feeding difficulties experienced by women taking part in a qualitative interview study of postnatal depression. Midwifery 20:251–260

Stampfer H G 1990 'Negative symptoms': a cumulative trauma stress disorder? Australian and New Zealand Journal of Psychiatry 24:516–528

Stanton J, Simpson A, Wouldes T 2000 A qualitative study of filicide by mentally ill mothers. Child Abuse & Neglect 24:1451–1460

Stevens A, Price J 1996 Evolutionary psychiatry: A new beginning. Routledge, London

Sullivan A, Raynor M, Oates M 2003 Why mothers die: perinatal mental health. British Journal of Midwifery 11:310–312

Tattan T, Tarrier N 2000 The expressed emotion of case managers of the seriously mentally ill: The influence of expressed emotion on clinical outcomes. Psychological Medicine 30:195–204

Tucker C, Barker A, Gregoire A 1998 Living with schizophrenia: caring for a person with a severe mental illness. Social Psychiatry and Psychiatric Epidemiology 33:305–309

Van Humbeeck G, Van Audenhove C, Pieters G et al 2001 Expressed emotion in staff-patient relationships: The professionals' and residents' perspectives. Social Psychiatry and Psychiatric Epidemiology 36:486–492

Vaughn C, Leff J 1976 The measurement of expressed emotion in the families of psychiatric patients. British Journal of Social Clinical Psychology 15:157–165

Vaughn C E, Leff J P 1981 Patterns of emotional response in relatives of schizophrenic patients. Schizophrenia Bulletin 7:43–44

Videbech P, Gouliaev G 1995 First admission with puerperal psychosis: 7–14 years of follow-up. Acta Psychiatrica Scandinavica 91:167–173

Viguera A C, Cohen L S, Baldessarini R J 2002 Managing bipolar disorder during pregnancy: weighing the risks and benefits. Canadian Journal of Psychiatry 47:426–436

World Health Organization 1992 The ICD-10 Classification of Mental and Behavioural Disorders: Clinical Descriptions and Diagnostic Guidelines. WHO, Geneva

Worsley A J 2000 Psychiatric disorders. In: Lee A, Inch S, Finnigan D (eds) Therapeutics in Pregnancy and Lactation. Radcliffe Medical Press, Abingdon, p 101–116

Zubin J, Spring B 1977 Vulnerability: A new view of schizophrenia. Journal of Abnormal Psychology 86:103–126

Chapter 7

Body image: change, dissatisfaction and disturbance

Victoria Lavender

INTRODUCTION

During pregnancy, women experience substantial changes in their body shape and weight that result in significant alterations of their body image, (Lederman 1984, Moore 1978, Strang & Sullivan 1985). Cash (1991) hypothesised that during pregnancy, because of the body changes that take place, women's appraisals of their bodies are activated. These appraisals draw upon currently held body image attitudes and ideas. Given the current western ideals about body shape, which suggest that thin women are more beautiful, desirable and socially admired, many pregnant women find themselves falling further from the cultural ideal of beauty. In this way, body image satisfaction may decline. The consequences of a negative body image may include such behaviours as dieting, starving or purging. This chapter will explore issues relating to levels of dissatisfaction with body image due to pregnancy and go on to explore the topic of eating disorders in which an excessive concern and dissatisfaction for body shape and weight and a disturbed perception of body image are part of the central criteria for diagnosis.

BODY IMAGE: CHANGE, SATISFACTION AND DISSATISFACTION

Body image, an internalised perception of the individual's own height, weight and shape is inevitably linked with self-esteem in which the individual evaluates her attractiveness, desirability and social worth or value. The cultural idealisation of female thinness (Garner & Garfinkel 1980) and the concomitant prevalence of body dissatisfaction, dieting, bingeing and purging among women

(Gilbert 1986, Grunewald 1985) and girls (Hill & Robinson 1991, Wardle & Marshland 1990) has been well documented. Indeed, dieting and an attendant diet mentality might now be described as both descriptively and prescriptively normative (Polivy & Herman 1987). However, an inaccurate or distorted perception of body image is not uncommon, particularly among women. Fallon and Rozin's (1985) study with college undergraduates demonstrated that a high percentage of young women perceived themselves far heavier than their actual size and therefore less attractive, than their male counterparts.

Generally, the expectation of weight gain during pregnancy is normalised, considered healthy and reinforced by social approval. Nonetheless, it can be presumed that for some women, satisfaction with body image may further decline during their pregnancy. However, the evidence is not consistent. Goodwin et al (2000) reported a significant decline in body image from pre-pregnancy to early pregnancy, while Richardson (1990) found that women viewed the bodily changes of pregnancy as transient and 'unique to childbearing endeavour' and went on to report that women were able to assimilate these changes without distress. Indeed, Davies & Wardle (1994) found in women attending antenatal clinics, the pregnant role conferred respectability to weight gain that would otherwise be unacceptable. These women were more accepting of their larger body size and less distressed than they anticipated in the early part of the pregnancy. The study by Boscaglia & Skouteris (2003) indicates that pregnant women who exercised for at least 90 min/week of moderate intensity activity expressed significantly greater satisfaction with body image at 15–22 weeks' gestation compared with low exercising pregnant women.

Perhaps the evidence of satisfaction in the postpartum period presents even greater ambiguities. While Mercer (1981), Wood Baker et al (1999) and Jenkins & Tiggemann (1997) all suggest that body image dissatisfaction intensifies in the postpartum period, Strang & Sullivan (1985) found that women were more satisfied with the shape of their bodies 6 weeks postpartum compared with during late pregnancy. In the Boscaglia study, both high and low exercising groups predicted some degree of dissatisfaction with body image postpartum, confirming the suggestion of Davies & Wardle (1994) that following the birth the pressure to achieve and maintain a thin figure is likely to be reinstated.

Jordan et al (2005) rightly urge caution in interpreting evidence of dissatisfaction with body image postpartum without full consideration of the contexts of the expressed dissatisfaction. The variability in the research may reflect incongruence in terms of the questions posed or the participant samples used, for example whether the women were primigravid or multigravid and whether 2 weeks or 12 months postpartum. Equally significant is that much of the research fails to explore the complexities and variability of women's individual narratives of new motherhood. In their research, a number of distinctive narratives emerge but body image was of variable importance and not prioritised over narratives, including those reflecting family support, the degree of stress experienced or missing personal space.

Concerns with body shape and weight might be viewed in wider contexts including those of health. Devine et al (2000) suggest that pre-pregnancy orientation towards weight emerged as the main influence on attitudes towards weight, diet and exercise behaviour during pregnancy and postpartum. Lips (1985) reports that physical stress might be of greater concern postpartum than body image. Kline et al (1998) conclude that while body image and weight gain concerns were expressed in both positive and negative terms, these were among a range of other concerns which can be grouped into four key domains: physical (e.g. pain, fatigue), psychological (e.g. depression), sexual (e.g. functioning and satisfaction) and social (e.g. confidence in parenting).

Relationship with the fetus

Body image during pregnancy is influenced by the way in which women conceptualise and represent their relationship with their fetus. The experience of pregnancy, with all the physical and emotional changes involved raises questions for women about their sense of identity and embodiment. Lupton (1999) presents these questions as: 'Is the fetus part of one's body/self, or is it separate? Where do I, the woman, begin, and it, the fetus end? How much control do I have (if any) over this fetus as it grows inside my body? How much control does it have over me?' The majority of the research concerning the relationship between a pregnant woman and her unborn baby has tended to focus on questions of the nature of attachment in relation to the development of maternal behaviours and attitudes following the birth.

Rubin (1984) identifies the 'separating out' of mother and baby into individual bodies/selves as a specific developmental task of women during pregnancy. Rubin describes a woman's sense of a symbiotic 'unity in wholeness and oneness' during the first two trimesters of pregnancy. During this period, it is difficult for women to determine 'what is self and what is baby – what happens to self also happens to baby'. Rubin proposes that it is only in the last trimester of pregnancy that a woman develops a sense of boundary between herself and the child, a 'separating out' from the psychological and physical unity of pregnancy.

Ballou (1978), Lumley (1980, 1982), Cranley (1981) and Stainton (1990) present four distinctive phases in women's developing awareness of the fetus; incorporating the fetus into the body and self image, differentiation of the fetus from self, gaining a sense of the child and finally attachment. There is an emphasis on the importance and the need for women to move through these stages progressively in their efforts to resolve the questions concerning identity and embodiment.

However, Schmied & Lupton (2001) argue that this view, commonly held in the theoretical and empirical literature of the relationship between the mother and her unborn child, as a progressional developmental process, might be challenged. In their study, the experience of the women's relationship was ambiguous and uncertain. Despite the tangible evidence, by late pregnancy, of their swollen abdomen and other bodily changes, experiencing the movements of the fetus and seeing it on ultrasound, the women found it difficult to come to terms with the fact that there was indeed a separate body within their own, which would soon emerge and have its own autonomous embodiment and identity. Sandelowski & Black (1994:610) describe the way in which both men and women 'tacked back and forth throughout the pregnancy and in the immediate post delivery period from the child in the head, to the child in the womb, to the child on the screen and to the child they anticipated in their arms'.

Schmied & Lupton argue that the notion of a progressive and orderly development of the emergence of the unborn child's identity is heavily influenced by a masculine and clinically based perceptual framework, in that it ignores the more ambiguous and fluid experiences of pregnant women: 'the shifting and fluid nature of the female body, including the capacity to reproduce another body within itself and to feed an infant via breast milk, suggests a multiplicity of ways of being that go beyond the limited nature of the masculinised ideal subject' Schmied & Lupton (2001:38).

Perhaps the ambiguities and somewhat contradictory nature of the evidence relating to changes and satisfaction in body image discussed earlier might also transmit to the questions generated in women's relationship to the unborn child. If the relationship between mother and child does not necessarily follow the developmental stages of identity separation that Rubin and others propose, but fluctuates and changes in a more fluid manner, perhaps the concerns voiced by women on the dissatisfaction of body image echo some of the ambiguities of the nature of identity and autonomy. Voicing concerns of the fetus as 'alien' to the body, particularly under the pressures of the anticipated and perhaps more socially acceptable emotional responses expected by others within the dominant discourse of the 'contented and happy' mother, may be verbalised in more generalised concerns of changes of shape and weight. Negative body image, a tangible and measurable concept, could include the less easily verbalised and intangible epistemological concerns of pregnant women.

This area of enquiry clearly warrants further study. The focus on clinical or care-related aspects of pregnancy, in which important dimensions of women's embodied experiences are often given less prominence, fails to address these important issues. Understanding pregnancy and the relationship between a mother and baby as dynamic and changing is likely to challenge previous understandings of the development of maternal–fetal attachment. Recognising that many women find it hard to conceptualise a body image of the fetus as distinct and separate from their own bodies/selves questions the orthodox view that good mothering depends on the successful and complete separation or individuation by birth or early in the postpartum period.

EATING DISORDERS

Although women's dissatisfaction with body image is not in itself an uncommon phenomenon, a distorted perception of body image, an excessive concern with shape and weight and eating behaviours such as self-induced vomiting, purging and severe dietary restraint or restriction are commonly indicators of an eating disorder. The clinical features of anorexia nervosa and anorexia bulimia will be discussed before exploring how these disorders may impact upon pregnancy.

A description of anorexia nervosa by the physician Louis-Victor Marcé in 1860 astutely illustrates many of the difficulties still to be faced by today's healthcare professionals when caring for a client with this complex and disabling disorder:

'We see . . . young girls, who at the period of puberty and after a preco-
cious physical development, become subject to inappetency carried to the
utmost limits. Whatever the duration of their abstinence, they experience
a distaste for food, which the most pressing want is unable to overcome;
. . . these patients arrive at a delirious conviction that they cannot or
ought not to eat . . . the affective sentiments undergo alteration . . . these
unhappy patients only regain some amount of energy in order to resist
attempts at alimentation, and very often the physician beats a retreat
before their desperate resistance'.

(cited in Silverman 1989:833–834).

It is suggested that women with an ongoing eating disorder have
been estimated to represent 1–6% of all women (Turton et al 1999).
The incidence rates of anorexia nervosa are highest in women
between the ages of 15 and 19 years old. This is estimated by
Turnbull et al (1996) to be 10 times higher in women than men and
Lucas et al (1999) note an upward trend in incidence since the early
1950s. Bulimia nervosa is more commonly seen and occurs in a
wider age range of women with a peak onset occurring between
the ages of 20–24 years. In addition to anorexia nervosa and bulimia
nervosa, two further classifications, binge eating disorder and
eating disorder not otherwise specified are included in the DSM
-IV (American Psychiatric Association, APA 2000). Further diagnostic categories have been proposed, including multi-impulsive
bulimia, to address clients with eating disordered and comorbid
personality disorder traits and machismo nervosa, to address a primarily male preoccupation with weight training and muscle gain.
The diagnostic criteria are shown in Boxes 7.1 and 7.2.

It is important to stress that many clients do not fulfil the full criteria for a diagnosis of anorexia or bulimia and that perhaps it may
be useful to conceptualise eating disorders as lying on a continuum with the likelihood of overlapping and changing symptoms
(Kornstein & Clayton, 2002).

There is clear evidence of the comorbidity of eating disorders and
depression. Casper (1998) estimates a lifetime prevalence rate of
major depression in anorexia nervosa of 46–74% in the restricting
type, and 46–80% in the binge-purge type. A less severe form of
depression, known as dysthymia, has overall lifetime prevalence in
anorexia nervosa of 19–93%. In bulimia nervosa, major depression
has a lifetime prevalence of 50–60% and the prevalence of
dysthymia ranges between 6–95%. Anxiety and eating disorders
are also closely connected. Godart et al (2000) report a lifetime

Box 7.1   Diagnostic criteria for anorexia nervosa – DSM-IV

1. Refusal to maintain body weight at or above a minimal normal weight for age and height (that is, weight <85% of that expected, or failure to make expected weight gain during a period of growth leading to body weight <85% of that expected).
2. Intense fear of gaining weight or becoming obese, even though the person is underweight.
3. Disturbed experience of the person's own body weight and shape.
4. In females who have experienced menarche, absence of three or more consecutive menstrual cycles, or the occurrence of periods only after hormone administration.

In addition, the type of anorexia is specified. In the restricting type, the person has not regularly engaged in binge eating or purging and utilises dieting, fasting and/or exercise to lose weight. In the binge eating/purging type, the person regularly engages in binge eating or purging, for example self-induced vomiting, misusing laxatives, enemas or diuretics.

Box 7.2   Diagnostic criteria for bulimia nervosa – DSM-IV

1. Recurring episodes of binge eating (characterised by consumption of large quantities of food in a discrete time period and a sense of losing control over eating during the episode).
2. Recurring compensatory behaviours to prevent weight gain included self-induced vomiting; misusing laxatives, enemas, or diuretics, or other medications; fasting or exercising excessively.
3. The binge eating and compensatory behaviours both occur at least twice weekly for 3 months on average.
4. Self-evaluation is excessively influenced by body weight and shape.
5. The disorder does not occur exclusively during episodes of anorexia nervosa.

There are two types of bulimia nervosa: the purging type (in which self-induced vomiting or misuse of medication occurs) and the non-purging type (in which other inappropriate compensatory methods are used, such as over-exercising or fasting).

prevalence of anxiety and anorexia nervosa of 83% and 71% in bulimia nervosa with social phobia as the most common presentation of anxiety.

The physical consequences of anorexia nervosa are that individuals are emaciated and often have cold, blue extremities. Some have signs which are secondary to the low intake of food, namely constipation, low blood pressure, bradycardia, sensitivity to cold and hypothermia. Amenorrhoea and subsequent fertility problems are common. Vomiting and the abuse of laxatives may lead to alkalosis and hypokalaemia and these abnormalities may cause epilepsy or, rarely, death from cardiac arrhythmia.

The physical consequences of bulimia nervosa are largely as a result of repeated vomiting. Potassium depletion is particularly serious, resulting in weakness, cardiac arrhythmia and renal damage. Urinary infections, swollen parotid glands, tetany, menstrual irregularities and epileptic seizures may also occur. There may be considerable damage to the teeth caused by the repeated vomiting of acid gastric contents. The individual with bulimia is likely to be of normal weight as excessive exercising, vomiting or purging prevents any weight gain as a consequence of binge eating.

Norman & Ryrie (2004) suggest that people with anorexia nervosa have an almost ten-fold risk of dying compared with healthy people the same age and sex and that the mortality rate from anorexia nervosa is the highest of any psychiatric illness. According to James (2001), the mortality rate for bulimia nervosa is approximately 7% for those with a 5-year history of the disease. In studies undertaken where the cause of death is specified (for example Herzog et al 2000), 54% of the subjects died as a result of eating disorder complications, 27% committed suicide and the remaining 19% died of unknown or other causes.

While there is evidence that the prevalence of eating disorders seems to have arisen over the past 30 years (Russell 1995), the aetiology remains both inconclusive and controversial. Most of the research over this time (see Szmukler et al 1995 for a review) tends to fall into two major categories; aetiological theories and maintenance models. Aetiological risk factors concerning the development of an eating disorder tend to be clustered around dieting, weight and eating. These include a family history of obesity in binge eating and bulimic disorders (Fairburn et al 1997, 1998) and a family history of leanness in anorexia nervosa (Hebebrand & Remschmidt 1995). General predisposing risk factors include sexual and physical abuse and neglect (Johnson et al 2002) and insecure attachment patterns in early psychological development (Ward et al 2001).

The risk factors that may maintain or perpetuate an eating disorder include negative self-belief; feelings of worthlessness, uselessness, inferiority, being a failure, fears of abandonment and fears of being alone (Cooper et al 1998). Stice (2002) points to interpersonal and relationship difficulties, the pursuit of perfectionism and the internalisation of the thin idealised body shape.

In exploring the aetiology and risk factors associated with the development and maintenance of an eating disorder, Goss & Gilbert (2002) suggest that a functional analysis, involving the careful and detailed exploration of the client's perception of the function they ascribe to their own behaviour, can give important information on the role that an eating disorder has for that individual and thus an insight into what it might feel like to experience such a disorder. Serpall et al (1999) note that for some individuals, their eating disorder had become a 'friend' in terms of helping them to feel protected, special and in control. The function of self-starvation or overeating for Orbach (1979) is self punishment and the avoidance of intimacy. For Cooper et al (1998) the function of an eating disorder enables a diversion from overwhelming emotional difficulties arising from adverse early experiences.

Goss & Gilbert (2002) explore the role that body shame and pride have in the development and maintenance of disordered eating behaviour; areas that only recently have been granted any degree of attention. They argue that for some individuals, particularly those who restrict their diets, body shame can arise out of a general sense of personal shame and inferiority where changing body shape and controlling desires (such as eating) are seen as solutions. Moreover, they can feel proud of themselves (and at times superior to others) when they control their eating behaviour and weight. The ability to resist their own desires and the influence/control of others can be built into their identity. For those who overeat and/or binge, eating behaviours can be used to distract the self from shame and negative feelings in general, but lead in the longer term to feelings of more shame. This sets up a vicious cycle where behaviours that help control feelings, of unworthiness for example, increases overall shame and thus poor eating control.

Specific areas of shame in eating disorders may include shame of the body shape and size. This can lead to excessive body monitoring (mirror-checking, or pinching parts of the skin as a 'fat test'), prompting feelings of self disgust or loathing and renewed attempts to control dietary intake. Alternatively, individuals may take great pains to avoid seeing their own body (or have others seeing it) in order to avoid body appearance shame. Some obese clients report avoiding mirrors, glass doors and windows in case they inadvertently see their reflection. Many report that they avoid public exposure of their bodies, (e.g. in fitness or gymnasium centres, swimming pools or communal changing rooms).

Body shame may also relate to body function, for example in sexual behaviour, sexual expression or the fear of impotence. Bulimics and individuals who binge, report shame following periods of excessive eating. Anorexic individuals also report shame when they have eaten very small amounts of food; they are likely to feel betrayed by their bodies' need to eat and feel disgusted by the food they are ingesting. Shame can be induced by the use of diuretics, laxatives or vomiting. Hiding these behaviours is common; this is likely to be motivated by fears of shaming responses by other people if they were to be discovered.

Perhaps one of the most common experiences for clinicians working with clients with eating disorders is the client's denial of their difficulties, particularly in the early phases of an eating disorder. Goss & Gilbert (2002) suggest that one way of making sense of denial in the face of the client's emaciation, or unmistakable evidence of bingeing behaviour, is to see this in terms of trying to cope with the stigma and shame associated with having a psychiatric diagnosis. Unhappily, the individual with an eating disorder is beset by the difficulties associated with their avoidance of belonging to one socially undesirable group (the overweight) by engaging in behaviour that places them in another stigmatised group (the mentally ill).

There is a clear danger of over generalisation in trying to provide a summary of how an individual might feel in having an eating disorder, for much will depend on the nature of the disorder and the behaviours adopted in order to manage the difficulties. However, common experiences include panic and extreme anxiety at losing control over idealised weight or shape, shame and distress in attempting to manage both the fear of social rejection of the coping mechanisms themselves; starvation, vomiting, purging or binging and the shame of the stigma of a psychiatric diagnosis.

To date, according to Norman & Ryrie (2004), there is very little evidence to support the efficacy of treatment interventions in primary healthcare settings. Indeed the study by Turnbull et al

(1996) indicates that 80% of cases of anorexia nervosa and 60% of bulimia nervosa are referred on for specialised help. However, since the publication of the National Service Framework (Department of Health, DoH 1999) a number of health authorities have produced care pathways for eating disorders, which may increase confidence in primary healthcare professionals to treat the less severe presentations of these disorders. In addition, The National Institute for Clinical Excellence Guidelines (NICE 2004) for eating disorders recommend that GPs take responsibility for the initial assessment and the initial coordination of care which will include the determination of the need for emergency medical or psychiatric assessment.

Until very recently, in-patient treatment for anorexia nervosa was regarded as standard, particularly if a high medical risk was strongly indicated. Clinical examination should include body mass index (BMI, calculated as body weight in kg divided by height in m^2), muscle strength and blood pressure, pulse rate, temperature and circulation. The practice guidelines recommended by the American Psychiatric Association for admission to hospital are when body mass index <16 kg/m^2 or weight loss >20%. In the UK, the current admission criteria is approximately <65% of the expected standard weight. The NICE guidelines recommend that most clients with anorexia nervosa should be managed on an out-patient basis unless there is a marked deterioration or a lack of significant improvement necessitating more intense monitoring and treatment, or where there is a significant risk of suicide or self harm.

According to the NICE guidelines, the broad aims of treatment should be to 'reduce risk, to encourage weight gain and healthy eating, to reduce other symptoms relating to an eating disorder, and to facilitate psychological and physical recovery' (NICE 2004: 1.2.2.3). A weight gain of 0.5–1 kg per week is recommended for anorexia nervosa clients in in-patient settings and a weekly gain of 0.5 kg for those in an out-patient setting. This requires approximately 3500 to 7000 extra calories a week. Feeding against the will of the client is only done as a last resort but can be administered under the current mental health legislation, such as the Mental Health Act 1983 or the Children Act 1989.

Therapies recommended to be considered for psychological treatment of anorexia nervosa include cognitive analytical therapy (CAT), cognitive behaviour therapy (CBT), interpersonal psychotherapy (IPT), focal psychodynamic therapy and family interventions focused explicitly on eating disorders. There is a very limited evidence base for the pharmacological treatment of anorexia nervosa and caution in prescribing antipsychotic medication and tricyclic antidepressants is necessary, particularly in view of the compromised cardiovascular function of many clients with anorexia nervosa.

In-patient treatment is rarely necessary for the treatment and care for clients with bulimia nervosa and the great majority of clients can be managed safely as out-patients. There are, however, some particular circumstances in which risk issues, such as self harm or suicide, or medical comorbidity such as diabetes mellitus may warrant a short admission as an in-patient. A specifically adapted cognitive behaviour therapy for bulimia nervosa (CBT-BN) is recommended by the NICE guidelines (2004) and confirmed by Hay & Bacaltchuk (2000) as effective. Unlike the treatment recommended for anorexia nervosa, antidepressant therapy and specifically selective serotonin reuptake inhibitors (SSRIs), for example fluoxetine, are the drugs of first choice in terms of acceptability, tolerability and reduction of symptoms.

EATING DISORDERS AND PREGNANCY

This chapter will now consider anorexia nervosa and bulimia nervosa in relation to pregnancy. Undisclosed eating disorders as the result of an individual's reluctance or shame in disclosing problems around food and eating behaviour may make the detection of eating disorders in pregnant women very difficult. Although perhaps it is unlikely that a midwife will see an obstetric client in a state of advanced starvation, it is highly likely that pregnant women with eating disorders are seen and will actively engage in food restriction, purging, binging and vomiting behaviour. The impact of eating disorders on fertility and pregnancy outcome will now be considered.

In the past, it was believed that pregnancy in women with anorexia nervosa was rare, primarily because of the endocrinological, psychological and psychosocial features of the disorder. Many women with anorexia nervosa have amenorrhoea, are sexually inactive and have an increased rate of fertility problems (Patel et al 2002). However, where this is not the case, studies by Kohmura et al (1986) and Bulik et al (1999) indicate that long-term fertility may not be compromised. Although many women with anorexia nervosa believe that amenorrhea protects them against pregnancy, this is not the case, as Mitchell-Gieleghem et al (2002) note, the absence of menstruation does not necessarily mean the absence of ovulation.

In Abraham's study (1998) of sexuality and reproduction of 48 women with a 10–15 year history of bulimia nervosa, amenorrhea was common (81%) and 63% of those studied were without their menstrual periods for more than 12 months. Bulimia clients are more likely to be of normal weight and be sexually active; therefore, the pregnancy rate is likely to be higher. Morgan et al (1999) found higher rates of oligomenorrhoea in their sample of women with bulimia nervosa and reported that 75% of pregnancies were unplanned because menstrual irregularities were (incorrectly) believed to imply infertility.

A number of case studies have suggested that eating disorders during pregnancy place both the mother and unborn child at risk (Crow et al 2004, Franko et al 2001, Kouba et al 2005) and this is exacerbated when the eating disorder is undisclosed or where an underlying eating disorder is overlooked. Maternal complications that have been noted in women with anorexia nervosa when compared with healthy women include a higher rate of miscarriage and a higher likelihood of caesarean deliveries (Bulik et al 1999, Franko et al 2001). Mitchell et al (1991) report high caesarean rates in women with bulimia nervosa. It is not clear why the caesarean rate among women with eating disorders is significantly higher. Contributory factors may include nutritional compromise during the gestational period, fetal abnormalities, or fetal malpresentation. Franko & Spurrell (2000) suggest that women with an active eating disorder may be identified as high risk by healthcare professionals, which may increase the probability of caesarean birth. For women with bulimia nervosa there are reports of excessive weight gain and the further risk of complications such as preeclampsia and hypertension (Bulik et al 1999, Fairburn & Welch 1990).

Behaviours that are characteristic of eating disorders, such as low pre-pregnancy weight and low weight gain during pregnancy, are associated with low infant birth weight, (Abrams & Laros 1986, Bulik et al 1999, Conti et al 1998, Waugh & Bulik 1999) low APGAR scores, a higher occurrence of breech presentation, and cleft lip and palate, (Conti et al 1998, Peterson et al 2004, Treasure & Russell 1988). In a control study by Kouba et al (2005), 49 nulliparous nonsmoking women, previously diagnosed with eating disorders, were shown to have delivered infants with a significantly lower birth weight, smaller head circumference and a greater risk of small for gestational age (SGA) and microcephaly.

Not all studies confirm the risks associated with pregnancy and a pre-existing eating disorder. For example, Steiner et al (1991) found no difference in maternal pregnancy weight gain and infant birth weight in their sample of mothers with anorexia nervosa compared with controls. Lemberg et al (1992) in a similar manner reported normal birth weight in children of the mothers with eating disorders in their sample. What seems to be fairly uncontroversial is the view from Namir et al (1986) that neither the occurrence of pregnancy complications nor the rate of birth defects exceeded that of the general population, when women with anorexia gained adequate weight throughout their pregnancy.

Less research has been undertaken on the impact of pregnancy on eating disorder symptoms. Mitchell-Gieleghem et al (2002) suggest that pregnancy can exacerbate both symptoms of anorexia nervosa and bulimia nervosa. However, Abraham (1998) notes that in her study with women with bulimia a proportion of the women demonstrated short-term episodes of bulimic-free behaviour with a marked reduction in vomiting, purging and binging. This is confirmed by Crow et al (2004) who note a significant reduction in binge eating and purging, particularly in the use of laxatives, but found that few women in their study were able to abstain entirely from their usual eating patterns. Fairburn et al (1992) also found reduction in restrictive eating behaviour and fewer episodes of over eating.

The underlying reasons for the suggestion of symptom improvement in eating disorders during pregnancy are by no means clear. One can speculate that a desire to protect the fetus or not harm the baby might mediate improvement, that although the mother might feel they do not 'deserve' to eat, the baby does. This rationale might allow the legitimisation of less restrictive eating patterns of anorexia nervosa or less reliance on strict methods of weight control associated with bulimia nervosa during the gestational period.

Lemberg & Phillips (1989) found in their clinical sample of women with eating disorders, the fear of losing control over weight gain was the single most prevalent anxiety during pregnancy. The majority of mothers did not confide their eating disorders to their obstetricians and had particularly strong negative reactions towards weighing. Most of this sample of women voiced concerns over the possibilities of physical damage to the unborn child as a result of their poor nutrition.

The postpartum period would appear to represent a particularly vulnerable time for the exacerbation of eating disorder patterns of behaviour. Stein & Fairburn (1996) found that eating disorder symptoms returned to a greater intensity than before pregnancy, markedly increasing at 3 months postpartum, and then plateaued at 6 months postpartum. Lemberg & Phillips (1989) found that half the women who had made a significant improvement in their eating disorder behaviour during their pregnancy actually relapsed in the first year after birth. Morgan et al (1999) found that in their study of 94 women with bulimia nervosa, the majority of the sample relapsed in the first 12 months postpartum, with over half experiencing more severe symptoms than before pregnancy. Relapse was predicted by unplanned pregnancies, symptoms of bulimia nervosa in the second trimester, previous history of anorexia nervosa, gestational diabetes and postnatal depression. Women who relapsed also had a lower BMI, more binges at conception, and greater alcohol consumption.

Several studies have examined breast-feeding patterns in women with eating disorders. Foster et al (1996) together with Barnes et al (1997) found that women's attitudes towards their bodies predicted intention to breast-feed. Those with high body shape and weight concerns were less likely to breast-feed their infants and this was further associated with low fetal attachment status during pregnancy. Insufficient lactation and allergies or negative reactions to breast milk are reported by Evans & Grange (1995). Waugh & Bulik (1999), Stein & Fairburn (1989), Lacey & Smith (1987) and Larsson & Andersson-Ellström (2003) all report that women with eating disorders had considerably more difficulty maintaining breast-feeding and resorted to bottle feeding in the early weeks of the postpartum period.

Perhaps it is not surprising that infant feeding problems associated with mothers with an eating disorder have been reported to persist throughout the infant and toddler years. Stein et al (1994) in a 1-year observational case-control study of 1-year-old children of primigravid mothers with eating disorders, found that these mothers were significantly more likely than controls to express negative comments towards the infant at meal times, but not during play, suggesting some specific influence of the eating disorder on parenting at mealtimes. There was more conflict at mealtimes between the mothers with eating disorders and their children than for the control group. Mothers with eating disorders were more intrusive, cutting across and/or disrupting the child as well as missing the child's cues.

Case studies from Russell et al (1998) and Fahy & Treasure (1989) report that some mothers with bulimia nervosa have difficulties in feeding their children, and often do not keep food in the house, while those with anorexia nervosa are more likely to underfeed their children, in a variety of ways, ranging from dilution of bottle feeds in early childhood, to reducing the overall amount of food available, confining food to mealtimes, forbidding sweets and discouraging children's requests for second helpings in later childhood. Reassuringly, Waugh & Bulik (1999) in a series of small case studies involving mothers with anorexia and bulimia nervosa found no gross deficiencies in the diets of infants aged 1–4 years old. Nevertheless, Stein et al (1994) found that at 12 months of age, the infants of mothers with eating disorders weighed less than controls.

The most significant predictor of weight at 12 months was conflict between mothers and infants observed at mealtimes; when mother–infant interaction was relatively smooth and harmonious the infants were likely to be heavier, but when it was more conflictual the infants were likely to be lighter. Stein et al (1996) examined whether parents with eating disorders misjudge their children's size or want them to be thin and thus limit their food intake. However, they discovered that mothers with eating disorders did not prefer thinner babies nor did they misperceive their 1-year-old children's size. In fact, these women were highly sensitive to their children's body shape and were accurate at judging their children's size and weight. What this would seem to indicate is that misperception of body size and shape is confined to the individual's own body image and is not applied to others, including their children.

Almost all the research to date has concerned mothers with eating disorders. Very few studies have examined fathers with eating disorders or included the roles and attitudes of fathers in exacerbating, ameliorating, or acting independently of the possible influences of a mother who has an eating disorder. This makes it all the more important that caution is advised in extrapolating the evidence concerning mothers with eating disorders to the future development of eating disorders of their children. Park et al (2003) point to a number of mechanisms which may mediate any influence parental eating disorders have on child development. First, genetic influence has been shown to play a role in this area, but much of the research remains inconclusive regarding the extent and nature of genetic influences. Second, parental psychopathology may impinge directly on the child; some parents have been shown to withhold or restrict food, as they do for themselves. It is not clear as yet whether this has a long-term detrimental effect upon the child in early or later years.

Third, the quality of parenting, in the role conflict has between the mother with eating disorder and the child may have a significant effect upon later psychological development; conflict at mealtimes may influence the child's food intake and, equally important, their perception of food as enjoyable and acceptable. Fourth, the question of role modelling and learnt behaviour must also be considered in assessing the reasons for any future development of eating disorders. Parents with eating disorders may act as poor role models for children in relation to eating behaviours and attitudes, either through dieting or their own eating behaviours.

THE ROLE OF THE MIDWIFE

A number of authors (Franko & Spurrell 2000, Morgan 1999, James 2001) have emphasised the need for a multidisciplinary team to help the obstetrician treat the pregnant women with an eating disorder; the role of the midwife is less well explored. The National Institute for Clinical Excellence (NICE) guidelines for eating disorders may encourage further expansion of the role of the midwife by recommending that 'pregnant women with eating disorders require careful monitoring throughout the pregnancy and in the postpartum period' (NICE 2004:1.1.4.4). In addition, it is likely that midwives will contribute to meeting the guideline 'pregnant women with either current or remitted anorexia nervosa should be considered for more intensive prenatal care to ensure adequate prenatal nutrition and fetal development' (NICE 2004:1.2.4.7).

Given the reluctance of many women to disclose their eating disorder and the shame associated with the stigma of a diagnosis of mental disorder discussed earlier, it is possible that in the monitoring of prenatal weight gain, the midwife may suspect or detect eating problems that have remained hidden for some time. It is possible that pregnant women with an eating disorder will reveal their distress more clearly during the process of being weighed. Asking the client how they would prefer to be weighed, whether for example, they would like to be offered the opportunity to step backwards onto the scales so that they do not visualise their weight, or how they would like to be told of weight gain; if they choose to be told at every visit or at pre-planned selected points during the pregnancy, it may help to reduce or at least not add unnecessarily to feelings of panic or distress. A planned weight gain regime, one that has been agreed in collaboration with the client and all members of the clinical and medical team, is recommended by Mitchell-Gieleghem et al (2002) as it offers the client the opportunity for the continuation of a sense of control over dietary intake.

The importance of sensitive, warm and non-judgemental interpersonal communication between the midwife and women with an eating disorder cannot be over emphasised. It is particularly important to appreciate that feelings associated with losing control and the resultant panic arising out of weight gain and the alteration of body image may result in increased eating disordered behaviour as the individual desperately seeks to regain a sense of control through restrictive dietary intake, purging, vomiting or binging.

The midwife needs to bear in mind that for persons with an eating disorder, food is a means by which feelings are controlled or smothered, only to be replaced by additional feelings of guilt and possibly shame. Well-meaning and enthusiastic comments on weight gain during pregnancy can be misinterpreted as negative reinforcements of an already low self-esteem. Positive comments such as 'that's good, you have gained a kilogram', aimed at encouraging a less restrictive nutritional intake or a reduction in binging or purging, may be misinterpreted as, 'you have gained a kilogram which is proof that you are a bad and despicable person'.

The midwife must aim to establish a collaborative partnership with the client by limiting their comments on weight to the links between maternal weight gain and fetal well-being and thereby providing a constructive rationale for the alteration of previously held patterns of eating. Mitchell-Gieleghem et al (2002) suggest that fetal models, which illustrate the size and development of the fetus, can be used to promote positive nutritional behaviours by the mother without overwhelming the client with feelings of guilt.

Dietary advice alone, unless given in conjunction with psychosocial support and appropriate psychotherapy and given by personnel with specialist knowledge of eating disorders, is likely to be ineffective and even counterproductive. A number of authors, including Brinch et al (1988), Mitchell-Gieleghem et al (2002) and Patel et al (2002) agree that collaboration with a dietician skilled in the management of eating disorders is essential, in order to incorporate as many of the women's food preferences and rituals as possible, increases adherence to the recommendations and provides feelings of security in a fear-provoking situation.

Close monitoring of the mother throughout the pregnancy involving tests for serum electrolytes, blood urea nitrogen, serum creatinine and an electrocardiogram, is necessary. Correction of metabolic imbalance and dehydration are vital. Clients with anorexia nervosa can display a low-normal T4, decreased T3 and a normal thyroid-stimulating hormone. Significant weight loss or failure to adequately increase weight; potassium levels <2.5 mmol/L, accompanied by electrocardiogram changes, indicate the need for admission. Cardiac enzyme changes or acute abdominal symptoms require immediate attention (Mitchell-Gieleghem et al 2002).

Following the pregnancy, it is vital to provide close postpartum supervision. The comorbidity of depression and anxiety with eating disorders, together with sleep deprivation, difficulties in breastfeeding and parenting a newborn for the first time or adjusting to an expanded role as a parent of a second or third child, may combine to present a period of extreme psychological difficulty. It has been described earlier that a sense of a loss of control in this period and efforts to regain the sense of coping and therefore control through well-established patterns of restricted dietary intake, purging, vomiting or binging can propel mothers into a severe relapse of eating disorder symptoms. The close interprofessional partnership between the midwife, obstetrician, nutritionist and, wherever possible, members of the eating disorders specialist service, in forging a collaboration with women with eating disorders is absolutely essential if they are to receive the appropriate care and support they need for themselves and for their infant.

CONCLUSION

The role of the midwife in caring for women with eating disorders is one that presents considerable challenges but also considerable key opportunities in the contribution to positive fetal and maternal outcome. Further research on the role of the midwife in the care of the client with an eating disorder is needed in order to determine the most effective interventions and care strategies that might be used with this client group.

References

Abraham S 1998 Sexuality and reproduction in bulimia nervosa patients over 10 year. Journal of Psychosomatic Research 44:491–502

Abrams B, Laros R J 1986 Prepregnancy weight, weight gain, and birth weight. American Journal of Obstetrics and Gynaecology 154:503–509

American Psychiatric Association (APA) 2000 Diagnostic and statistical manual of mental disorders (DSM-IV TR), 4th edn. American Psychiatric Press, Washington

Ballou J W 1978 The Psychology of pregnancy. Lexington Books, Lexington, MA

Barnes J, Stein A, Smith T et al 1997 Extreme attitudes to body shape, social and psychological factors and reluctance to breastfeed. Journal of the Royal Society of Medicine 90:551–559

Boscaglia N, Skouteris H 2003 Changes in body image satisfaction during pregnancy: A comparison of high exercising and low exercising women. Australian and New Zealand Journal of Obstetrics and Gynaecology 43:41–45

Brinch M, Isager T, Tolstrup K 1988 Anorexia nervosa and motherhood: Reproduction pattern and mothering behaviour of 50 women. Acta Psychiatrica Scandinavica 77:611–617

Bulik C, Sullivan P, Fear J et al 1999 Fertility and reproduction in women with a history of anorexia nervosa: A controlled study. Journal of Clinical Psychiatry 60:130–135

Cash T F 1991 The treatment of body image disturbance. In: Thompson J (ed.) Body image, eating disorders, and obesity: an integrative guide for assessment and treatment. American Psychological Association, Washington, p 83–107

Casper R C 1998 Depression and eating disorders. Depression and Anxiety 8(suppl 1):96–104

Conti J, Abraham S, Taylor A et al 1998 Eating behaviour and pregnancy outcome. Journal of Psychosomatic Research 44:465–477

Cooper J M, Todd G, Wells A 1998 Content, origins and consequences of dysfunctional belief in anorexia nervosa and bulimia nervosa. Journal of Cognitive Psychotherapy 12:213–230

Cranley M S 1981 Roots of attachment. The relationship of parents with their unborn. Birth Defects Original Article Series xvii:59–83

Crow S J, Keel P K, Thuras P et al 2004 Bulimia symptoms and other risk behaviors during pregnancy in women with bulimia nervosa. International Journal of Eating Disorders 36:220–223

Davies K, Wardle J 1994 Body image and dieting in pregnancy. Journal of Psychosomatic Research 38:787–799

Department of Health (DoH) 1999 National service framework for mental health: modern standards and service models. DoH, London

Devine C M, Bove C F, Olson C 2000 Continuity and change in women's weight orientations and lifestyle practices through pregnancy and the postpartum period: the influence of life course trajectories and transitional events. Social Science and Medicine 50:567–582

Evans J, Grange D 1995 Body size and parenting in eating disorders: A comparative study of the attitudes of mothers towards their children. International Journal of Eating Disorders 18:39–48

Fahy T, Treasure T 1989 Children of mothers with bulimia nervosa. British Medical Journal 299:1031

Fairburn C F, Welch S L 1990 The impact of pregnancy on eating habits and attitudes to shape and weight. International Journal of Eating Disorders 9:153–160

Fairburn C G, Doll H A, Welch S L et al 1998 Risk factors for binge eating disorder: a community based case-control study. Archives of General Psychiatry 55:425–432

Fairburn C G, Stein G, Jones A R 1992 Eating habits and eating disorders during pregnancy. Psychosomatic Medicine 54:665–672

Fairburn C G, Welch S L, Doll H A et al 1997 Risk factors for bulimia nervosa. A community based case-control study. Archives of General Psychiatry 54:509–517

Fallon A E, Rozin P 1985 Sex differences in perceptions of desirable body shape. Journal of Abnormal Psychology 94:102–105

Foster S F, Slade P, Wilson K 1996 Body image, maternal fetal attachment and breastfeeding. Journal of Psychosomatic research 4:181–184

Franko D, Blais M A, Becker A E et al 2001 Pregnancy complications and neonatal outcomes in women with eating disorders. American Journal of Psychiatry 158:1461–1466

Franko D, Spurrell E 2000 Detection and management of eating disorders during pregnancy. Obstetric Gynecology 95:942–946

Garner D, Garfinkel P 1980 Socio-cultural factors in the development of anorexia nervosa. Psychological Medicine 10:647–656

Gilbert S 1986 Pathology of eating: psychology and treatment. Routledge, London

Godart N T, Flament M F, Lecrubier Y et al 2000 Anxiety disorders in anorexia nervosa and bulimia nervosa: co-morbidity and chronology of appearance. European Journal of Psychiatry 15:38–45

Goodwin A, Astbury J, Meeken J 2000 Body image and psychological well-being in pregnancy. Australian and New Zealand Journal of Obstetrics and Gynaecology 40:442–447

Goss K, Gilbert P 2002 Eating disorders, shame and pride: a cognitive-behavioural functional analysis. In: Gilbert P, Miles J (eds) Body shame: conceptualisation, research and treatment. Brunner-Routledge, London, p 219–255

Grunewald K K 1985 Weight control in young college women: who are the dieters? Journal of the American Dietetic Association 85:1445–1450

Hay P J, Bacaltchuk J 2000 Psychotherapy for bulimia nervosa and binging. The Cochrane Database of Systematic Reviews 4:CD000562

Hebebrand J, Remschmidt H 1995 Anorexia nervosa viewed as an extreme weight condition: genetic implications. Human Genetics 95:1–11

Herzog D B, Greenwood D N, Dorer D J et al 2000 Mortality in eating disorders: a descriptive study. International Journal of Eating Disorders 28:20–26

Hill A J, Robinson A 1991 Dieting concerns have a functional effect on the behaviour of nine year old girls. British Journal of Clinical Psychology Review 9:393–407

James D C 2001 Eating disorders, fertility and pregnancy: relationships and complications. Journal of Perinatal and Neonatal Nursing 15:36–48

Jenkins W, Tiggemann M 1997 Psychological effects of weight retained after pregnancy. Women and Health 25:89–98

Johnson J G, Cohen P, Kasen S et al 2002 Childhood adversities associated with risk for eating disorders or weight problems during adolescence or early childhood. American Journal of Psychiatry 159:394–400

Jordan K, Capdevila R, Johnson S 2005 Body or beauty: a Q study into post pregnancy body image. Journal of Reproductive and Infant Psychology 23:19–31

Kline C R, Martin D P, Dayo R A 1998 Health consequences of pregnancy and childbirth as perceived by women and clinicians. Obstetrics and Gynaecology 92:842–848

Kohmura H, Miyake A, Aono T et al 1986 Recovery of reproductive function in patients with anorexia nervosa: A 10 year follow up study. European Journal of Obstetrics, Gynecology and Reproductive Biology 22:293–296

Kornstein S G, Clayton A H 2002 Women's mental health. Guildford, New York

Kouba S, Hällström T, Lindholm C et al 2005 Pregnancy and neonatal outcomes in women with eating disorders. Obstetrics and Gynecology 105:255–260

Lacey J, Smith G 1987 Bulimia nervosa: The impact of pregnancy on mother and baby. British Journal of Psychiatry 50:777–781

Larsson G, Andersson-Ellström A 2003 Experiences of pregnancy-related body shape changes and of breast-feeding in women with a history of eating disorders. European Eating Disorders Review 11:116–124

Lederman R P 1984 Psychosocial adaptation in pregnancy: assessment of seven dimensions of maternal development. Prentice Hall, Englewood Cliffs, New Jersey

Lemberg R, Phillips J 1989 The impact of pregnancy on anorexia and bulimia nervosa. International Journal of Eating Disorders 8:285–295

Lemberg R, Phillips J, Fischer E 1992 The obstetric experience in primigravida anorexic and bulimic women – some preliminary observations. British review of Bulimia and Anorexia Nervosa 6:31–38

Lips H M 1985 A longitudinal study of the reporting of emotional and somatic symptoms during and after pregnancy. Social Sciences and Medicine 21:631–640

Lucas A R, Crowson C S, O'Fallon WM et al 1999 The ups and downs of anorexia nervosa. International Journal of Eating Disorders 26:397–405

Lumley J 1980 The image of the fetus in the first trimester. Birth and the Family Journal 7:5–14

Lumley J 1982 Attitudes to the fetus among primigravidae. Australian Paediatric Journal 18:106–109

Lupton D 1999 Risk and the ontology of pregnant embodiment. In: Lupton D (ed.) Risk and socio-cultural theory: new directions and perspectives. Cambridge University Press, Cambridge

Mercer R T 1981 The nurse and maternal tasks of early postpartum. American Journal of Maternity and Child Nursing 6:341–345

Mitchell J E, Seim H C, Glotter D et al 1991 A retrospective study of pregnancy in bulimia nervosa. International Journal of Eating Disorders 10:209–214

Mitchell-Gieleghem A, Mittelstaedt M E, Bulik C M 2002 Eating disorders and childbearing: concealment and consequences. Birth 29:182–191

Moore D S 1978 The body image in pregnancy. Journal of Nursing and Midwifery 22:17–27

Morgan J F 1999 Eating disorders and reproduction. Australian and New Zealand Journal of Obstetrics and Gynaecology 39:167–173

Morgan J F, Lacey J H, Sedgwick P M 1999 Impact of pregnancy on bulimia nervosa. British Journal of Psychiatry 174:135–140

Namir S, Melman K, Yager J 1986 Pregnancy in restrictor-type anorexia nervosa: A study of 6 women. International Journal of Eating Disorders 5:837–845

National Institute for Health and Clinical Excellence (NICE) 2004 National clinical practice guideline: eating disorders: core interventions in the treatment and management of anorexia nervosa, bulimia nervosa, and related eating disorders. NICE, London

Norman I, Ryrie I 2004 The art and science of mental health nursing. Open University Press, Maidenhead

Orbach S 1979 Fat is a feminist issue. Hamlyn, London

Park R J, Senior R, Stein A 2003 The offspring of mothers with eating disorders. European Child and Adolescent Psychiatry 12:111–119

Patel P, Wheatcroft R, Park R et al 2002 The children of mothers with eating disorders. Clinical Child and Family Psychology Review 5:1–19

Peterson Sollid C, Wisborg K, Hjort J et al 2004 Eating disorder that was diagnosed before pregnancy and pregnancy outcome. American Journal of Obstetrics and Gynecology 190:206–210

Polivy J, Herman C P 1987 Diagnosis and treatment of normal eating. Journal of Consulting and Clinical Psychology 55:635–644

Richardson P 1990 Women's experiences of body change during normal pregnancy. Maternity and Child Nursing Journal 19:93–111

Rubin R 1984 Maternal identity and the maternal experience. Springer, New York

Russell G F M 1995 Anorexia through time. In: Szmukler C, Dare C, Treasure J (eds) Handbook of eating disorders. John Wiley & Sons, Chichester, p 5–18

Russell G F M, Treasure J, Eisler I 1998 Mothers with anorexia nervosa that underfeed their children: their recognition and management. Psychological Medicine 28:93–108

Sandelowski M, Black B P 1994 The epistemology of expectant parenthood. Western Journal of Nursing Research 16:601–622

Schmied V, Lupton D 2001 The externality of the inside: body images of pregnancy. Nursing Inquiry 8:32–40

Serpall L, Treasure J, Teasdale J et al 1999 Anorexia nervosa: Friend or foe? International Journal of Eating Disorders March 25:177–189

Silverman J A 1989 Louis-Victor Marcé, 1828–1864: Anorexia nervosa's forgotten man. Psychological Medicine 19:833–835

Stainton M C 1990 Parent's awareness of their unborn infant in the third trimester. Birth 17:92–96

Stein A, Fairburn C G 1989 Children of mothers with bulimia nervosa. British Medical Journal 299:777–778

Stein A, Fairburn C G 1996 Eating habits and attitudes to body shape and weight in the postpartum period. Psychosomatic Medicine 58:321–325

Stein A, Murray L, Cooper P et al 1996 Infant growth in the context of maternal eating disorders and maternal depression: a comparative study. Psychological Medicine 26:569–574

Stein A, Woolley H, Cooper S D et al 1994 An observational study of mothers with eating disorders and their infants. Journal of Child Psychology and Psychiatry 35:733–748

Steiner H, Smith C, Rosenkranz R T et al 1991 The early care and feeding of anorexics. Child Psychiatry and Human Development 21:163–167

Stice E 2002 Risk and maintenance factors for eating pathology: A meta-analytic review. In: Norman I, Ryrie I 2004 The art and science of mental health nursing. Open University Press, Maidenhead

Strang V R, Sullivan P L 1985 Body image attitudes in pregnancy and the postpartum period. Journal of Obstetric and Gynaecological Neonatal Nursing 14:332–337

Szmukler C, Dare C, Treasure J (eds) 1995 Handbook of eating disorders. John Wiley & Sons, Chichester

Treasure J L, Russell G F M 1988 Intrauterine growth and neonatal weight gain in babies of women with anorexia nervosa. British Medical Journal 296:1038

Turnbull S, Ward A, Treasure J et al 1996 The demand for eating disorder care. An epidemiological study using the general practice research database. British Journal of Psychiatry 169:705–712

Turton P, Hughes P, Bolton H et al 1999 Incidence and demographic correlates of eating disorder symptoms in a pregnant population. International Journal of Eating Disorders 25:123–133

Ward A, Ramsey R, Turnbull S et al 2001 The adult attachment interview in anorexia nervosa: A transgenerational perspective. British Journal of Medical Psychology 74:497–505

Wardle J, Marshland L 1990 Adolescent concerns about weight and eating: a social developmental perspective. Journal of Psychosomatic Research 34:377–391

Waugh E, Bulik C M 1999 Offspring of women with eating disorders. International Journal of Eating Disorders 25:123–133

Wood Baker C W, Carter A S, Cohen L R et al 1999 Eating attitudes and behaviours in pregnancy and postpartum: global stability versus specific transitions. Annals of Behavioural Medicine 21:143–148

Chapter **8**

Substance misuse and mental health

Victoria Blunsden, Sian Monahan and Stephanie Withers

INTRODUCTION

Substance misuse is a major problem facing our society today, with the prevalence of recreational drug abuse among young people having increased markedly over the past two decades (Krzysztof & Kuezkowski 2003). However, when a pregnant woman misuses drugs, both she and her unborn child may suffer harm (Walker 1999). In addition, substance misuse often creates or is accompanied by an array of social problems for the user and those around her, including violence, child abuse and neglect, and family dysfunction (Haack 1997). Harm to children born of substance-using mothers can be far-reaching, affecting both their physical and cognitive growth and development and there are numerous obstetric complications arising from drug abuse in pregnancy (Bertis et al 2003). In addition, it is acknowledged in the Confidential Enquiry into Maternal and Child Health that 8% of all women who died were substance misusers, representing an almost trebling of reported deaths from the last triennium (NICE 2004).

This chapter will examine the theories of addiction, the effects of substance misuse in pregnancy, dual diagnosis and treatments available. Consideration will also be given to the care that can be provided by the multidisciplinary team.

THEORIES OF ADDICTION

To demonstrate a broad understanding of the concept of drug dependence in pregnancy, it is essential that it is explored in relation to some of the theories of addiction. 'Addiction' is a commonly understood word to use with respect to excessive appetite behaviours and is described as 'a compulsive physiological and psychological need for a habit-forming substance' (Webster 1998). However, the experience of being an addict is less widely understood, with substance misusers rarely receiving the public sympathy or understanding that other groups who live with debilitating conditions do.

There are many theories of addiction to underpin substance misuse. However, it is essential that they are understood because each theory suggests a different treatment or approach to helping women who have drug-related problems. This will enable the practitioner to work from a more considered viewpoint and engage the correct professional groups and agencies, thereby enhancing multi-professional and multi-agency involvement.

The moral model

Moral models are based on beliefs or judgements of what is right or wrong, acceptable or unacceptable. What these judgements imply are that people who use drugs are bad or sinful and this offers no real help to overcome their addiction. The 'treatment' under this model tends to be punishment. Unfortunately, this model remains a powerful influence on a minority of health and social care professionals. A punitive attitude may deter the pregnant women from accessing antenatal care or fail in keeping them within the service (Craig 2001). This puts both the pregnant woman and her baby at risk. Since women may be fearful of the reaction of health workers to their pregnancy, the care provided should be non-judgemental and supportive.

Biological models

This model implies that women addicted to drugs have a biological abnormality that causes them to become addicted. It is similar to the moral model in the fact that it is perceived there is something wrong with the individual, rather than that they have an illness. It is believed that there is an individual biochemical interaction between a person and a substance and that this has a connection with addictive behaviour. Evidence also exists that some, but not all, addicted people have an inherited predisposition towards substance dependency (Petersen & McBride 2004). According to this model, addictions are incurable diseases and the best that can be hoped for is to achieve remission through abstinence. Both pharmacological and behavioural treatments are used. The most common of these are methadone programmes and motivational therapy/12-step programmes. The western approach to addiction is centred on these biological theories, and the rapid advances in genetic exploration and neuropsychopharmacology are enabling a better understanding and treatment of addictions (Petersen & McBride 2004).

Personality model

Theories of personality as a cause of addictive behaviour lie some-where between the biological and the psychological models. The expression 'addictive personality' is often used, but it is argued that there is no one type of personality more likely to become dependent on drugs (Nathan 1988). Nevertheless, substance misuse has been linked with aspects of personality such as antisocial personality, some characteristics of personality disorders, risk taking, novelty seeking and reward dependency (Otter & Martin 1996).

Psychological models

There are many different psychological theories that can be applied to a substance misuser but the main view of these theories is that the addiction is a behaviour problem. Under these models the user is not bad or deficient but has become addicted because of the processes that take place within a person's mind. The addiction can also be as a result of how a substance affects our bodies and minds, and anyone can be affected because of these reasons. Pregnancy offers a unique opportunity to intervene with women who have substance misuse disorders, since their motivation to change their drug use behaviour may be greater due to their concern for the baby. With this in mind, increasing the woman's motivation to change her drug habit could be achieved through motivational interviewing.

Social learning model

Social learning is a psychological model of understanding drug addiction, developed by Bandura (1977). This theory has three aspects, the first is that drug use is learned and continues because there is a desired outcome from its use. Second, using drugs is learnt in response to certain stimuli – people, places, things, events, thoughts and feelings. The final aspect is self-efficacy when a person recognises the negative effects of using drugs but does not feel capable of change, so is unlikely to try.

Sociological model

This model examines the influence that tension, guilt, stress, aggression and conflict can have on the use of drugs. It is perceived that the primary role of the use of drugs is to reduce anxiety. Another suggestion is that some societies produce a higher level of these emotions and are permissive of/or encouraging drug use. This model also examines the influence of those who stand to make a profit from selling the drugs. Treatment would involve changing our society and although such efforts can have an impact, sociological change happens over time and therefore will be too slow a process to be of immediate help to the pregnant woman (McMurran 1994).

DRUGS AND ALCOHOL IN PREGNANCY

The prevalence of women's substance misuse in pregnancy within the UK is difficult to predict, due to the difficulties in collecting information and the problems which women have in disclosing their drug/alcohol use. Regional figures from the south west of England have indicated that prevalence in women who disclose that they are misusing substances during pregnancy is approximately 1% for drug use and 4% for alcohol drinking (BMDS 2005). Research looking specifically at women drug users entering treatment, found that 90% were of childbearing age (Gossop et al 1998).

The risks to the fetus of taking both legal and illicit substances during pregnancy are well documented, and include intrauterine growth retardation (IUGR), placental abruption, miscarriage, premature labour and delivery and fetal alcohol syndrome (Sprauve et al 1997). It should be noted however, that the effects of individual substances are difficult to measure precisely, due to the multifactorial confounding factors associated with substance misuse (Bertis et al 2003).

During pregnancy, the main focus is generally on fetal health, but women who use substances suffer higher morbidity and mortality rates and their health is frequently compromised due to the lifestyles and risky behaviour which taking substances entails.

Women who are drug dependent are often poly-drug users, putting their bodies through a physiological challenge when they combine vasoconstrictive drugs such as cocaine and amphetamine, with sedative drugs such as heroin, benzodiazepines and alcohol. Society as a whole has a poor view of women who use drugs and alcohol in pregnancy, and women often face stigmatisation from their own families, peers and professionals, which may prevent them accessing care (Drummond & Fitzpatrick 2000).

It is important that pregnant substance-misusing women are regarded as pregnant women who have a drug problem, rather than drug users who happen to be pregnant. The impact on pregnancy will depend on the drugs used and the presence of other medical or social problems (Craig 2001). If there are significant problems with the drug use, particularly if the women have chaotic lifestyles, then there are increased rates of perinatal morbidity and mortality with poorer maternal health. Therefore, drug-using women have potentially high-risk pregnancies and require comprehensive multi-professional care, which will ensure mental, medical and social problems are all addressed.

Why do women use drugs/alcohol in pregnancy?

Women entrenched in drug taking or alcohol drinking behaviour, often have histories of sexual abuse, physical abuse, rape and domestic violence, and take refuge in substances as a coping mechanism (Becker & Duffy 2002). The lifestyle of the chaotic polydrug user is a cycle of scoring the drug, funding their habit through stealing, sex work or borrowing, using the drug and dealing with the effects. Normality as most people know it ceases to exist within their lives, and many years may pass whereby this lifestyle becomes the norm. Consequently, when women become pregnant, and choose to commence a methadone maintenance programme, although they may be adults, they do not have the emotional maturity which one would expect from their peers, since a large portion of their lives, sometimes from early teenage years, has been taken up using substances. Anecdotally, women give complex reasons for their substance misuse, for example (BMDS 2005):

> 'My dad sexually abused me when I was 13; one day, my friend gave me some gear (heroin) and I felt OK, it made it go away, so it's his fault that I started on it'.

> *Polydrug user aged 22*

'All of my friends did it (crack), so I smoked some to be the same. I don't do it all of the time, and I'm not addicted like . . . to the Gear, I can stop whenever I want, but it's hard 'cos crack makes me feel really good. When I think back, I know I was really stupid to start doing it, I had no problems like some people have when they start using'.

Polydrug user aged 29

'I used to smoke cannabis from when I was about 15, then I met my boyfriend who was using gear, and I started it too. I'm clean now, but it's still really hard as he's still doing it and on bad days I still want to, but I don't'.

Ex user aged 20

How do women feel about their use during pregnancy?

Pregnant women misusing substances often feel guilt regarding continued usage and the effects of the drugs on their unborn baby. Unfortunately, although they may have the best of intentions, most women are drug dependent and stopping is often easier said than done. Many women express concerns regarding methadone in pregnancy, as they fear that their baby will be born dependent, failing to recognise that many of their babies are already dependent on heroin. Women may say that they want to stop using substances, but the reality is that many will not be at the stage of their lives when they are ready to stop. Pregnancy forces the issue to become a major factor in their lives, which previously they may not have addressed or intended to address. However, pregnancy can also act as a motivator to the women to change their lives, since most women will put the needs of their families and unborn baby above their own (NICE 2004).

Women may also have a fear of engaging in maternity services, as they fear their baby will be removed and taken into care (Thomson & Green 1996). Some women have previous experience of social services, and may have a child or children that have been removed from them. A subsequent pregnancy may reawaken feelings of grief over the removal of their child/children and make them reluctant to access maternity services. Those that do access maternity services will almost certainly have social services involvement, and they may spend their entire pregnancy worrying about what will happen to their unborn baby.

Child protection concerns

Many will question the addict's ability to care for her baby. However, dependence per se affords insufficient grounds to separate mother and baby (Llewelyn 2000). Substance misuse by a parent should not automatically indicate child neglect or possible abuse (MacRory 1997). Indeed many women may view their pregnancy as an opportunity to change their lives, moving from chaos to stability during this period. However, the types of drugs used, along with the frequency and amount, may seriously impair the women's ability to safely parent their children, and increase the risk of other social problems such as domestic violence, frequent changes of accommodation, unsuitable childcare, and non-existent routine must be acknowledged (Kroll & Taylor 2003). Prentice & Watts (2004) suggest that it is a critical task for health professionals working with drug-dependant women to judge whether a child is suffering or likely to suffer harm. This may be problematic and it could be argued that automatic child protection registration is the safest option (Klee et al 2002). However, this discriminatory practice, or the assumption by women that it occurs, is the main reason why they are so fearful of social work intervention and should therefore be avoided (Prentice & Watts 2004). To overcome this, Klee et al (2002) suggest that working constructively with parents could improve the situation, with the social services contribution taking the form of family support rather than child protection (Petersen & McBride 2004).

PREGNANCY CARE AND MANAGEMENT

The Confidential Enquiry into Maternal and Child Health (NICE 2004) recommends that women who misuse substances should be managed within a wider multi-agency team, which includes both statutory and non-statutory agencies, following an integrated model of care. Pregnant drug users have many needs, and one service in isolation is not able to meet the needs of pregnant substance misusers. An integrated model of service seeks to meet the assessed needs of the individual, by combining services, forming partnerships and enabling the service user to access services formed within a 'one-stop-shop' approach. This type of approach is recommended due to the wide needs of service users, and includes drug treatment, family support, maternity services, social services and other agencies to meet the needs of the women and their families (National Treatment Agency 2002).

Women will often have complex social problems and may also be involved with the criminal justice system. Within the maternity services, it is often the role of the drug liaison midwife (specialist midwife) to liaise with other agencies in order to manage the women's care effectively. Women also need to be able to access maternity services and the wider multi-agency team as early as possible. This may mean booking women's pregnancies at 6 weeks' gestation, but this may ultimately improve outcomes for both the woman and her baby. The early engagement of women is advantageous since it gives both them and the multi-agency team an opportunity to develop a rapport which will increase the likelihood of women attending their appointments, and ensures that the team have ample opportunity to get to know the women well.

Drug-dependent women may be identified from any agency within the multi-agency team. They may be accessing other treatment services or women's groups and can be signposted to maternity drug services. Maternity services should have a robust referral system which will enable the women to access maternity drug services immediately. Alternatively, midwives may be the first person to whom the women disclose their drug use, at their pregnancy booking appointment, which is often extremely difficult for the women, as they fear they will be judged detrimentally. Routine questioning regarding drug use should be a part of the booking process, and approached as sensitively as possible. If midwives do not recognise the drugs that the women name, then they should ask the women for more information.

Following referral, women should be offered a clinic appointment with the wider multi-agency team, where they may be seen by each partner agency in order to assess their individual needs. The women should be offered a dating scan in the first instance to confirm pregnancy, since many women drug users suffer from amenorrhea and may not be pregnant. Confirmation of pregnancy enables the women to access maternity drug services where a needs assessment should be conducted, and the women can subsequently be directed to the services to suit her needs. During pregnancy, obstetric/midwifery management should have an holistic approach and should include:

- Consultant-led care
- Dating ultrasound scan

- Anomaly ultrasound scan
- Growth ultrasound scans at 28 and 32 weeks' gestation
- Screening for blood-borne viruses at booking and 3rd trimester
- Standard booking bloods
- Sexually transmitted infection screening at booking and 3rd trimester
- Nutrition
- Medical risk factors
- Drug/alcohol use
- Ongoing assessment regarding child protection concerns.

Fundamental to good care is that the management is based around a contract of care agreeable to all parties, where pregnancy is used as a window of opportunity to set harm-minimisation targets, not only to reduce the morbidity of pregnancy (NICE 2004), but also to provide a baseline for continued improved health in these susceptible women (Craig 2001).

TREATMENT OF DRUG AND ALCOHOL MISUSE IN PREGNANCY

Models of treatment may vary across the UK. This section describes the treatment options available to pregnant women with substance misuse problems, offered as part of an integrated multidisciplinary service in the south west of England (BMDS 2005).

The aim of prescribing a legal substitute for illicit drug use is to reduce the harm that illegal drug use causes the individual, to enable them to engage with their care plan, and in particular the psychological work necessary to help them make progress towards mutually agreed goals. Thus it is assumed that prescribing will always be delivered in the context of a therapeutic working relationship. The delivery of psychosocial interventions is an essential part of the complete treatment package, and prescribing without psychosocial interventions is largely ineffective (NTA 2004). Pregnant women should be prioritised for treatment and medication commenced as soon as possible, following a full assessment by a specialist drug service or GP shared care drugs worker. This should include the type of drugs, level, frequency, pattern, method of administration – and consider any potential risks to her unborn child from current or previous drug use. Women with more complex mental or physical needs, or those who are using drugs in a more chaotic, heavy manner, should ideally be managed by a specialist drug service and the GP should focus on managing the more stable client.

Opiates

If pregnant women are using opiates (such as heroin) on a daily and consistent basis, to such an extent that to cease using the drug would cause physical withdrawal symptoms, then substitute opiate prescribing is appropriate. This has the aim of offering stability to the woman and therefore the pregnancy, enabling the best possible outcome for mother and baby.

It is advisable, especially when tolerance is unknown, that on commencement of methadone or buprenorphine, the client should be seen daily for a few days. This allows the dose to be titrated to accommodate any withdrawal symptoms and avoid overdosing. This should also be the case when methadone is initiated in the maternity ward setting. Withdrawal symptoms can be difficult for women to deal with and should be recognisable to health professionals. Subjective and objective withdrawal symptoms include: craving for drugs, anxiety, drug seeking behaviour, hot and cold flushes, shivering, shaking hands, aching muscles and bones, reduced appetite, irritability, goose bumps (hence 'cold turkey'), and muscle twitching (hence 'kicking the habit'). In severe cases, there will be increased intensity of the above symptoms plus grossly disrupted or absent sleep, restlessness, stomach cramps, nausea, vomiting, diarrhoea, weakness, no energy, weight loss, slight pyrexia, spontaneous orgasm or ejaculation, increased respiratory rate and depth, tachycardia and raised blood pressure. Women may experience these feelings for some time if treatment is not titrated to their needs. The course of acute opiate withdrawal symptoms begins at 8–18 h for heroin and 24–72 h for methadone. The symptoms peak at 24–36 h for heroin and 36–72 h for methadone, and subside at 5–10 days for heroin and 2–3 weeks for methadone. See Table 8.1 for a description of objective withdrawal symptoms and dose titration. This may be particularly useful if a woman not previously in treatment is admitted to the ward, and it becomes clear at initial assessment that she has been using opiates.

Table 8.1 Severity of objective withdrawal

Signs[a]	Absent/Normal	Mild to moderate	Severe
Eyes watering	Absent	Eyes watery	Eyes streaming, wiping of eyes
Runny nose	Absent	Sniffing	Profuse secretion, wiping of nose
Agitation	Absent	Fidgeting	Cannot remain seated
Perspiration	Absent	Clammy skin	Beads of sweat
Goosebumps	Absent	Barely palpable, hairs standing up	Readily palpable, visible
Pulse rate (BPM)	<80	80–100	>100
Vomiting	Absent	Absent	Present
Shivering	Absent	Absent	Present
Yawning (>10 min)	<3	3–5	6 or more
Dilated pupils	Normal <4 mm	Dilated 4–6 mm	Widely dilated >6 mm

[a]Other objective signs can include raised blood pressure (BP), pallor, sneezing, leg cramps and stomach cramps.
(DoH et al 1999, Himmelsbach 1942, BMA 2002)

Opiate substitution

Methadone

Traditionally, methadone has been the drug of choice as it has been tried and tested for many years as the treatment for opiate addiction. It is long acting (24–36 h in the non-pregnant person) and is taken in oral liquid form so the consumption can be easily supervised by the pharmacist or nurse. It allows the client to move away from a drug using lifestyle (Table 8.2). It is possible to reduce methadone dose in pregnancy but this should be done gradually and by small amounts. It should be noted that due to increased metabolism and body tissue mass of the pregnant woman, the half-life of methadone can reduce to 10 h in the later stages of pregnancy. For this reason, it is advisable to split the methadone dose so that half is taken in the morning and half in the evening, from 20–28 weeks of pregnancy.

Some of the problems encountered with methadone treatment are due to the association the client has with it. It may have been prescribed for them in the past, with little success and therefore they have little faith in it. Some people report that it makes them feel sluggish and clouded. This feeling can serve a purpose for some clients in that it numbs their emotions allowing them to partially block painful memories in a similar way to illicit drug taking. Women often start using drugs in response to traumatic circumstances in their childhood and therefore find it difficult when exposed to emotions they may not have experienced for a long time. The other problem with methadone is the potential for opiate withdrawal in the neonate, which in some cases is quite severe and prolonged, probably due to the long half-life of methadone.

Buprenorphine

The alternative to methadone, and a drug that is relatively new in the treatment of pregnant women, is buprenorphine, also known as Subutex. This product was licensed in the UK for the treatment of opiate dependence in 1998, after studies found it to be less addictive than methadone and much safer in overdose (RCGP 2004). Buprenorphine is a mixed agonist-antagonist and its primary action is as a partial opiate agonist. Therefore, it reduces the impact of additional opioid use (when prescribed in doses >8 mg) by preventing the receptors being occupied by these additional opioids.

Table 8.2 Levels of tolerance

Categorisation of level of tolerance	Amount of heroin used over 24 h (indication of tolerance)	Initial dose of methadone to be given	Methadone dose increment given 4 hourly p.r.n. (if objective opiate withdrawal persists)
Low or uncertain	One £10 bag[a] or ¼ g	10–20 mg	5 mg
Moderate and high	≥2 × £10 bags[a] or ≥½ g	20–30 mg	10 mg

[a]A £10 bag of heroin typically contains 0.2 g heroin, but may contain as little as 0.1 g or as much as 0.3 g. Ask the client how much heroin is in the bag; the client will usually know.

The advantages of buprenorphine are that it is easier to reduce and come off, although this would still be done gradually in pregnancy and the withdrawal syndrome in the neonate is believed to be minimal.

This treatment is more appropriate for women who are ready and emotionally stable enough to feel their emotions, as they will most probably experience a clarity they have not felt for a while. This needs to be borne in mind and explained to the clients as they could find it difficult to manage painful or traumatic memories, which could result in relapse into drug use or other destructive behaviours such as self harm or eating disorders.

Detoxification

From opiates

Detoxification from opiates in the non-pregnant person is usually performed during a 2-week in-patient hospital stay or in the community over approximately the same length of time. Medication such as lofexidine can be given to enable the process to be less uncomfortable and distressing. Medication for symptomatic relief of insomnia, muscle aches and cramps can also be administered. However, in pregnancy, women would have to experience 'cold turkey' or acute withdrawal, which is very distressing and unpleasant. Therefore, detoxification from opiates during pregnancy should be avoided, but a gradual reduction in the dose over a number of weeks with the client controlling the reductions depending on how she is managing, both mentally and physically, may be offered. It may be beneficial to admit some women into hospital for a 1–2 week stabilisation period, particularly those who find it difficult to cease their illicit drug use. During this time, their medication can be adjusted accordingly to accommodate their 'on top' use. They can be carefully observed for any signs and symptoms of opiate withdrawal and the pregnancy may also be monitored.

From benzodiazepines

It is always difficult to ascertain the level of benzodiazepine dependency in pregnant women, as withdrawal could cause fitting. Benzodiazepines such as diazepam and nitrazepam are often bought illicitly on the street and consumed in large doses. Therefore, a careful drug history needs to be taken with particular detail as to how long the woman has been using, what happens if they do not use, and daily dosage (which is often vague). For those who are not prescribed benzodiazepines therapeutically, it is usual to start prescribing on a reducing basis in order to gradually detoxify them. If women wish to breast-feed once their baby is born, it is advisable to reduce the dose to a low level (below 15 mg daily). Benzodiazepines are usually reduced before methadone/buprenorphine.

From stimulants

Crack cocaine has been found to be used by 45% of pregnant women attending a maternity drugs service (BMDS 2005). Exposure to drugs such as cocaine and amphetamines are believed to be potentially damaging to the unborn baby (Slutsker 1992). Women should be advised to stop using these immediately. However, some women may find it very difficult to give up due to the changes that occur in the brain chemistry following long-term use. In-patient admission may be advantageous in allowing the woman a safe place to come off stimulants, while monitoring for any depression that may occur as a result.

From alcohol

Alcohol is considered potentially damaging to the unborn baby, and it is advisable for the alcohol-dependent pregnant woman to stop drinking (Beattie 1981). However, the sudden cessation of alcohol can result in withdrawal symptoms, (Box 8.1), some of which may be dangerous to both the mother and the unborn baby, depending on the level of physical dependence, Therefore, it is important that medical withdrawal of alcohol for the severely dependent pregnant woman is conducted in an in-patient setting, as there is the possibility of medical complications including grand mal fits.

The withdrawal process is managed by prescribing a benzodiazepine such as chlordiazepoxide or diazepam, although as with prescribing any medication in pregnancy, the risks versus the possible benefits of their use need to be assessed. Disulfiram (Antabuse) is contraindicated during pregnancy as its use has been associated with congenital abnormalities (Jessup & Green 1987). It is important to note that coming off drugs or alcohol in hospital may be undertaken relatively easily but it is remaining abstinent once discharged that is much more challenging.

Box 8.1   Symptoms of alcohol withdrawal

Early symptoms of alcohol withdrawal generally appear 6–48 h after drinking has stopped but can occur up to 10 days after the last drink. Withdrawal symptoms may include:

- Restlessness
- Tachycardia
- Irritability
- Hypertension
- Anorexia
- Insomnia
- Nausea
- Nightmares
- Vomiting
- Impaired concentration
- Sweating
- Impaired memory
- Tremor
- Elevated vital signs.

More severe symptoms of alcohol withdrawal may include:

- Increased tremulousness
- Increased agitation
- Increased sweating
- Delirium (with confusion, disorientation, impaired memory and judgement)
- Hallucinations (auditory, visual, or tactile)
- Delusions (usually paranoid)
- Grand mal seizures.

Note: Withdrawal symptoms do not necessarily progress from mild to severe. In some individuals, a grand mal seizure may be the first sign of withdrawal. Seizures usually occur 12–24 h after cessation or reduction of drinking. One-third of all patients who have seizures develop delirium tremens.

DUAL DIAGNOSIS

Studies have shown a correlation between childhood sexual abuse and mental health problems in later life, including anxiety, depression, self harm, eating disorders and borderline personality disorders (Roosa et al 1999). Substance misuse is sometimes used as a way of dealing with the pain of past trauma and temporarily serves a purpose for the woman, but when that behaviour stops, often other defence mechanisms or behaviours manifest themselves. Therefore, it is possible for a woman to deal successfully with drug using behaviour but then resort to self harm or bulimia for instance, while the underlying issues remain unresolved. The best scenario is to stabilise the woman in terms of medication and lifestyle in order for her to pursue therapy around her particular problem, which may involve referring her to another agency. Not all women are willing or able to confront their past, especially during pregnancy, as they may be feeling particularly vulnerable.

When the woman is diagnosed with a more severe and enduring mental health problem such as a psychotic illness, it is imperative for all agencies involved to liaise and have a clear plan and package of care. The complex combination of pregnancy, addiction and mental illness requires a carefully coordinated approach. These women are likely to be taking prescribed medication, such as antidepressants or antipsychotics, alongside their illicit drug or alcohol use, which may be contraindicated in pregnancy. The decision to continue or change medication needs to be addressed by the multidisciplinary team in conjunction with the obstetrician and psychiatrist. It must be remembered that evidence is inconclusive regarding the safe use of any psychotropic medication in pregnant women. Therefore, a thorough assessment of the risks versus the benefits must be made prior to administering these medications.

Stimulant drugs in particular can exacerbate underlying mental health problems and destabilise the mental state. The risk of using these drugs such as cocaine and amphetamine needs to be explained to the woman. If she is involved in chaotic illicit drug use, she may be less compliant in taking prescribed medication and therefore be vulnerable to relapse into psychotic symptoms.

The following general guidelines can be useful in assessing and managing the mental health of pregnant, substance-using women.

- Distinguish between drug-induced psychiatric symptoms and a major mental disorder. Some symptoms such as anxiety, agitation and paranoia can be due to drug intoxication or of the withdrawal syndrome itself. Therefore it should be established whether the client has used drugs and whether they have a history of mental illness. If necessary, ask the GP to arrange for a mental health assessment, or it may be possible for the specialist drug service to undertake this

- Establish communication early in treatment with the mental health personnel involved in the client's care. Permission to liaise should be sought from the client to obtain important information, which will help in the management of the client. Any information regarding risk assessment should be obtained at this stage. Careful planning of the in-patient stay should be considered along with management of any challenging behaviour
- Set up regular meetings to involve mental health workers, where appropriate, in monitoring the client's progress and treatment plan
- Consider child protection and social services involvement. There is an increased likelihood that a referral to a social worker would be undertaken to carry out an assessment due to the complexity of comorbidity. For those clients who are clearly psychiatrically unstable and using illicit drugs, parenting a baby may be unachievable.

CONCLUSION

It is evident that providing care to pregnant, addicted women requires the skills of a multi-professional team to provide all needed services, including appropriate treatment of drug problems. Assessments of appropriate treatment of psychosocial and mental health issues, as well as social services for the children also are essential. The multi-professional management team is clearly identified as involving midwives, including drug liaison midwife, obstetricians, social workers, drug teams and addiction units, and the care provided should be non-judgemental and supportive. This will increase the chances of a better outcome for mother and baby; both in the short and long term and Craig (2001) suggests that this will also achieve the aim of keeping women within the service, as a punitive attitude may deter those most in need of care.

However, it is clear that pregnant women who misuse illicit substances are at higher risk of obstetric complications and compromised babies and the overall aim of antenatal treatment varies according to the type of drug being used. It appears that further studies are required to determine the degree to which individual substances contribute to the associated obstetric complications and elucidation of those factors that may reduce this risk. Therefore, it is reasonable to assume that further research into drug dependency in pregnancy is necessary (Craig 2001).

Providing care for pregnant substance misusers gives rise to some acute ethical and legal dilemmas, but what is clear is that a balance is needed between the rights and needs of both mothers and babies. It would be irresponsible to ignore the possible risks of neglect and unrealistic to expect mothers to come for help if they are at risk of losing their children. The literature shows that many areas have a more therapeutic and less punitive approach to pregnant drug misusers (Siney 1999). Unfortunately, the low numbers of pregnant women attending drug agencies suggest that there is still much progress to be made.

References

Bandura A 1977 Social learning theory. Prentice-Hall, New York

Beattie J 1981 Fetal alcohol syndrome – The incurable hangover. Health Visitor 54:468–469

Becker J, Duffy C 2002 Women drug users and drugs service provision: service level responses to engagement and retention. DPAS Briefing Paper 17

Bertis B, Little B B, Snell L M et al 2003 Treatment of substance abuse during pregnancy and infant outcome. American Journal of Perinatology 20:255–262

Bristol Maternity Drugs Service 2005 Audit and outcomes 2004–2005. Unpublished report. BMDS Bristol

British Medical Association, Royal Pharmaceutical Society 2002 British national formulary. Pharmaceutical Press, UK

Craig M 2001 Substance misuse in pregnancy. Current Obstetrics and Gynaecology 11:365–371

Department of Health, Scottish Office Department of Health, Welsh Office, Department of Health and Social Services, Northern Ireland 1999 Drug misuse and dependence – guidelines on clinical management. HMSO, London

Drummond D C, Fitzpatrick G 2000 Children of substance misusing parents. In: Reder P, McClure M, Jolley A (eds) Family matters: interfaces between child and adult mental health. Routledge, London

Gossop M, Stewart D, Marsden J 1998 NTORS at one year. The National Treatment Outcome Research Study: changes in substance use, health and criminal behaviours one year after intake. DoH, London

Haack M R 1997 Drug-dependent mothers and their children. Issues in public policy and public health. Springer, New York

Himmelsbach C K 1942 Clinical studies of drug addiction – physical dependence withdrawal and recovery. Archives of Internal Medicine 69:766–772

Jessup M, Green J R 1987 Treatment of the pregnant alcohol-dependent woman. Journal of Psychoactive Drugs 19:193–203

Klee H, Jackson M, Lewis S 2002 Drug misuse and motherhood. Routledge, London

Kroll B, Taylor A 2003 Parental substance misuse and child welfare. Athenaeum Press, Gateshead

Krzysztof M, Kuezkowski M D 2003 Labour analgesia for the drug abusing parturient: is there cause for concern? Obstetric and Gynaecological Survey 58:599–607

Llewelyn R W 2000 Substance abuse in pregnancy: the team approach to antenatal care. The Obstetrician and Gynaecologist 2:11–15

MacRory F 1997 Standing Conference on Drug Abuse. Drug use, pregnancy and care of the newborn. Manchester

McMurran M 1994 The psychology of addiction. Taylor & Francis, London

Nathan P E 1988 The addictive personality is the behaviour of the addict. Journal of Consulting and Clinical Psychology 56:183–188

National Institute for Health and Clinical Excellence 2004 Confidential enquiry into maternal and child health. Why mothers die 2000–2002. Sixth annual report. NICE, RCOG Press, London

National Treatment Agency 2002 Models of care for the treatment of drug misusers. NTA, London

National Treatment Agency 2004 More than just a dose. NTA, London

Otter C, Martin C 1996 Personality and addictive behaviours. In: Bonner A, Waterhouse J (eds) Addictive behaviour: molecules to mankind. Perspectives on the nature of addiction. Macmillan, Hampshire

Petersen T, McBride A 2004 Working with substance misusers. A guide to theory and practice, 3rd edn. Routledge, London

Prentice S, Watts K 2004 Pregnant women and substance misuse: an audit. Journal of Midwifery 12:767–770

Roosa M W, Reinholtz C, Angelini P J 1999 The relation of child sexual abuse and depression in young women: comparisons across four ethnic groups. Journal of Abnormal Child Psychology 27:65–76

Royal College of General Practitioners 2004 Guidance for use of buprenorphine for treatment of opioid dependence in primary care. RCGP, London

Siney C 1999 Pregnancy and drug misuse. Midwives Press, London

Slutsker L 1992 Risks associated with cocaine use during pregnancy. Obstetrics and Gynaecology 79:778–789

Sprauve M E, Lindsay M K, Herbert S et al 1997 Adverse perinatal outcome in parturients who use crack cocaine. Obstetrics and Gynecology 89:674–678

Thomson B, Green A 1996 Services for women: the way forward. In: Harrison L (ed.) Alcohol problems in the community. Routledge, London

Walker J J 1999 Drug addiction in pregnancy. Contemporary Reviews in Obstetrics and Gynaecology 8:77–83

Webster M 1998 Marriam Webster's deluxe dictionary. Online. Available: http://www.m-w.com 11 April 2006

Chapter 9

Domestic abuse, violence and mental health

Kathleen Marion Baird

INTRODUCTION

The aim of this chapter is to discuss and bring attention to the magnitude of domestic abuse and the effect that domestic abuse can have on a woman's well-being and mental health. The chapter will examine the facts behind domestic abuse and discuss and deliberate the social context of domestic abuse. Domestic abuse and pregnancy will be examined where the role of the midwife and other health professionals in these areas will be explored. For the purpose of this chapter, the terminology of domestic abuse and domestic violence will be used interchangeably.

DOMESTIC VIOLENCE: THE FACTS

Domestic violence against women is a global health issue; this epidemic is widespread because it knows no boundaries; it extends across national, racial, cultural and economic factors. Therefore, the catastrophe of domestic abuse and more specifically the heartbreak of domestic abuse against women and girls will affect most people, at some point in their lives. This may occur directly as a result of a personal relationship, or through the occurrence of violence happening with close family members or friends. The ramifications of domestic violence are far reaching; violence against women is often a cycle of abuse that can transpire in many different types of abuse (Table 9.1) (World Health Organization 1997). Research has exposed strong associations between domestic violence and serious social, psychological and long-term health problems. Domestic abuse is not about an isolated case of aggression. It is often a pattern of behaviour that escalates over a period of time. It should be stressed

Table 9.1   Examples of violence against women throughout their life cycle

Phase	Type of violence
Pre-birth	Sex-selective abortion; effects of battering during pregnancy and birth outcomes
Infancy	Female infanticide; physical, sexual and psychological abuse; incest; child prostitution and pornography
Girlhood	Child marriage; female genital mutilation; physical, sexual and psychological abuse; incest; child prostitution and pornography
Adolescence and adulthood	Dating and courting violence (e.g. acid throwing and date rape) economically coerced sex; incest; sexual abuse in the workplace; rape; sexual harassment; forced prostitution and pornography; trafficking in women; partner violence; marital rape; dowry abuse; and murders; partner homicide; psychological abuse; abuse of women and disabilities; forced pregnancy
Elderly	Forced suicide or homicide of widows for economic reasons; sexual, physical and psychological abuse

World Health Organisation 1996 Violence against women, FRH/WHD/97.8:26–27

that any type of abuse does not have to occur regularly to generate an environment of trepidation and fear.

Domestic abuse places women and their children in danger in the very place where they should feel the safest: within a family environment in their home. For many women the home is often the place where they can feel most frightened and afraid at the hands of someone who is supposed to love and cherish them. Women who are victims of domestic abuse will suffer not only physically but also psychologically as they struggle to survive living with the ever-present threat of violence.

In recent years, there has been a greater understanding of domestic abuse, its causes and consequences. It has finally been realised that domestic violence against women is an abhorrent crime and infringement against their human rights. In some countries including the UK, domestic abuse is no longer considered a private matter between husband and wife, boyfriend and girlfriend. It is now being talked about in women's magazine's newspapers and television, and finally it has become the focus of Government policy. However, this has only come about because of the determined and untiring work of organisations such as Women's Aid who have campaigned with inexorable energy since the early 1970s to highlight the plight of women and their children as they attempt to survive living in a violent relationship.

Although there has been a wide and varied domestic violence discourse since the emergence of the very first woman's refuge in 1972, it is only recently that research, originating from Britain has focused specifically on the role that healthcare professionals can play in addressing domestic abuse. Researchers and health professionals are beginning to address the problem of domestic abuse because it has finally been realised that many women who experience domestic abuse will frequently use the health services as part of a wider help process (Stark & Flitcraft 1996). Progress continues to be slow in many areas; one suggestion for this could be that health professions are still attempting to define effective strategies to address domestic abuse.

UNDERSTANDING DOMESTIC VIOLENCE

It is vital to have an understanding of domestic violence before one can begin to understand how domestic violence can affect a woman's mental health and well-being. Previously, society was inclined to think of domestic abuse as a private matter between a couple that often resulted in a physical assault on a woman. This is partly due to the fact that physical assault is the most visible form of domestic violence, however in reality, domestic abuse can and does include several forms of abuse and in some relationships several different types of abuse can occur at the same time. This can include: sexual, emotional and psychologically abusive behaviours. There are several definitions of domestic violence, some of them describe the range of abusive behaviours that may be experienced, while others mention the relationship that exists between the victim and the perpetrator. Broadening the definition of domestic violence allows for the acknowledgment of not only physical, psychological and sexual violence but also the harm of living with threatening behaviour. One such inclusive definition is by the Government Domestic Violence Unit:

'Any incident of threatening behaviour, violence or abuse (psychological, physical, sexual, financial, or emotional) between adults who are or have

been intimate partners or family members regardless of gender or sexuality'.

(Department of Health 2005)

Prevalence and statistics of domestic violence

- The police in the UK receive a phone call for assistance with domestic violence every minute (British Crime Survey, Kershaw et al 2001)
- One woman is murdered every 3 days in England and Wales as a result of domestic violence (Home Office 1999)
- Women are the overwhelming majority of the most heavily abused group. Among people subjected to four or more incidents of domestic violence from a perpetrator, 89% were women (British Crime Survey, Kershaw et al 2001)
- Sexual victimisation affects 24% of women during their lifetime and for 17%, sexual victimisation has occurred since the age of 16 (British Crime Survey, Kershaw et al 2001)
- Maternal death through substance abuse is often associated with past and current experience of abuse with psychiatric or psychological problems which, while not constituting mental illness, cause major morbidity and contribute to death (Confidential Enquiry into Maternal and Child Health 2004).

Research shows that the vast majority of violence experienced by women occurs in the home, and that a husband or an intimate partner instigates it. However, it must be realised that other members of the extended family may also commit violence. A recent report conducted by John Hopkins University's population information programme ascertained that in over 50 population studies, domestic violence was occurring, and was therefore a serious human rights threat to all women in all societies, and that on average one in three women around the world has experienced violence in an intimate relationship (Heise et al 1999).

Current theoretical explanations

Theories drawn from academics and researchers suggest and trace domestic violence to causes such as personality disorders and interpersonal family dynamics, poverty and economic stress. Before developing an understanding of domestic violence and the devastating effect surviving daily with domestic violence can have on a woman's health and well-being, it is important to try to understand the context of domestic violence within society. Hoff (1990) proclaims that violence against women occurs in a climate of socially structured inequalities exemplified not only by the concept of patriarchy, but also sexism. Stark & Flitcraft (1996) would agree with Hoff (1990); they propose that previously little attention was paid to the interplay of macroevents such as equality and the microdynamics of male domination. In a social system where women's subordination to men is defined as natural, violence continues to be seen and accepted as a conventional means of controlling women. Dobash & Dobash (1979) discuss how violence can be seen as a result of conflict within a domestic relationship. They also believe that this relationship is based on the status and position of men in a patriarchal society. Four themes have been identified that exemplify conflict leading to domestic violence: men's possessiveness and jealousy; disagreements and expectations concerning domestic work and resources; men's sense of the right to punish their women for perceived wrong-doing; the importance to men of maintaining or exercising their power and authority. Their research highlighted the identifiable issues that may be a source of conflict and act as a trigger for violence to occur. These include:

- Domestic work
- Money
- Children
- Alcohol
- Possessiveness and jealousy
- Isolation
- Sex.

Presently, cultural explanations of domestic abuse emphasise the hierarchical implications of traditional sex and gender roles.

Rape and sexual abuse

The World Health Organization estimates that one in five women will suffer rape or attempted rape during their lifetime (Cebello et al 2004, Mooney 1993). Whatever the actual figures are, it can be assumed they are an underestimation. It is thought that any form of sexual violence perpetrated by a partner is universally under reported. In many countries, there has been little or no research carried out to investigate the problem. Indeed, in some countries sexual abuse and rape by an intimate partner is not considered a crime. There is an assumption that once a woman enters into marriage, the husband has the right to unlimited sexual access to his wife. Many women will choose not to disclose sexual abuse, due to the fear of reprisals from the perpetrator, or the worry of not being believed. Within the UK prior to 1991, the marital rape exclusion clause considered that rape in marriage could not happen and this allowed the spouse freedom from any criminal prosecution (Lees 2000).

Rape is a serious crime, whether it occurs inside or outside of a marriage or partnership. Reported rape incidents have increased by 165% in the last 10 years; this is a steeper rise than in any other form of crime (Home Office 1999), yet only 5.6% of rapes reported to the police currently result in a conviction (Amnesty International 2005). Rape is a crime, which, through fear, has a disproportionate impact on the way women live their lives. It is evident from a 5.6% conviction rate for reported rapes, that the Criminal Justice System in this country is failing rape victims.

Just as rape can occur between strangers, it also occurs between partners, friends and work colleagues. Pickup et al (2001) rightly proclaims that women never 'provoke' rape; it has to be realised that women's bodies are not the property of men and as such, they are free to consent to or refuse sex, inside as well as outside of a relationship. Coerced sex may result in sexual fulfilment for the perpetrator, however its main purpose is often an expression of power and control over the person being assaulted. Men who force or coerce a partner into a sexual act believe their behaviour is legitimate because they are married or cohabiting with the woman. In 2005, a UK-based poll carried out on behalf of Amnesty International showed widespread ignorance of the extent of rape and low conviction rates. However, what is more alarming is the belief that women themselves are to blame for being raped. A third (34%) of the people in the UK believe that a woman is partially or totally responsible for being raped if she behaved in a flirtatious manner. The poll also revealed that similar attitudes existed over clothing, drinking and whether a woman actually said (or meant) 'No' to the man (Amnesty International 2005). Clearly, these most recent findings expose a disquieting stance and attitudes towards women and a sexist blame culture.

Rape and sexual abuse is often believed to be carried out by strangers. However, for the majority of women who experience rape, they will actually know their attacker with many of them being a close relative, spouse, or acquaintance. When an assailant is a person who the woman has held in a position of love and trust, the abuse can lead to feelings of bewilderment and despair. Women are left feeling betrayed – not just by the men whom they trusted but by their own judgement. They are left feeling fearful of all men (Lees 2000).

Women who experience violence from their husbands and partners are 12 times more likely than other women to attempt suicide (Heise 1993). A cross-cultural study drawing on data from Africa and South America demonstrated that marital violence was a leading cause of female suicide (Pickup et al 2001). Rape and sexual violence have now been recognised as a tactic of repression and torture (Amnesty International 1991). Yet in spite of this, the rape and sexual assault of women continues; it often takes place on a massive scale in war and conflict where it is used to dominate, degrade and instill fear in women (Pickup et al 2001). There are many misconceptions about women and rape (Table 9.2). Rape and sexual violence has been associated with many mental health and behavioural problems in adolescence and adulthood. In one population-based study, the prevalence of women with a psychiatric disorder was 33% in women with a history of sexual abuse as an adult, 15% in women with a history of physical abuse carried out by an intimate partner and 6% in women who had not experienced any form of violence (Mullen et al 1988).

It has been reported that sexual abuse is often accompanied by physical and psychological abuse in violent relationships. It has been estimated that sexual abuse occurs in approximately 40% of all cases of domestic abuse (Campbell & Alford 1989). The physical consequences of rape include pregnancy, sexually transmitted disease and HIV. For some women who become pregnant as a result of rape, abortion may be objectionable to her on religious and cultural grounds.

THE PSYCHOLOGICAL EFFECTS OF DOMESTIC ABUSE ON WOMEN

The overall effects of living with domestic abuse are wide and varied, from physical injury, poor mental health, social isolation and overuse of drugs and alcohol as a means of escaping and coping with the abuse. The psychological effects of domestic violence can include depression, anxiety, post-traumatic stress disorder, flashbacks, nightmares, exaggerated startle response and suicide attempts (James-Hanman 1999). These feelings of low esteem will lead to a dependence upon the abuser. Findings from

Table 9.2   Myths and misconceptions about rape

Myth: rape occurs between strangers in dark alleys

Implications:

Assumes that nice girls do not get raped

Implies that the home is safe

Implies that rape can be prevented by avoiding certain places, and therefore blames the survivor

Assumes a particular survivor profile and therefore stigmatises her

Entrenches, racial and class prejudices

Facts:

More than half of all rapes were committed by persons known to the survivor

Date rape is very common

Women are often raped in their own homes

Myth: Women provoke rape by the way they dress or act

Implications:

Attempts to excuse rape and blame the survivor

Assumes that a woman who draws attention is looking for sex or 'deserves' what she gets'

Stigmatises the survivor

Facts:

Dressing attractively and flirting are an invitation for attention, and/or admiration, not for rape

Only the rapist is responsible for the rape!

Myth: Rape is a crime of passion

Implications:

Assumes that rape is impulsive and unplanned

Assumes men to be incapable of controlling sexual urges

Assumes that rape is about uncontrollable lust

Attempts to excuse, minimise and romanticise rape

Facts:

Research evidence from rapists themselves suggests that most rapes are premeditated and planned

Most rapists failed to get an erection or ejaculate

Interviews with rapists reveal that they rape to feel powerful and in control, not for sexual pleasure

Many rapists are involved in sexually satisfying relationships with wives or girlfriends at the time of the rape

Stereotypically 'unattractive' women are raped; this includes the elderly and young children

Myth: If she did not scream, fight, or get injured, it was not rape
Implications:
  Disbelieves and traumatises the survivor
  Invalidates her experience
  Discourages her from seeking help

Facts:
  Women in rape situations are afraid of being killed or seriously
    injured, and cooperate with the rapist to save their lives
  Rapists use many manipulative techniques to intimidate and
    coerce women
  Women in a rape situation often become physically paralysed
    with terror or shock, and are unable to move or fight
  Non-consensual intercourse does not always leave visible signs
    on the body or the genitals

Myth: You can tell if she has 'really' been raped by how she acts
Implications:
  Disbelieves and re-traumatises the survivor
  Invalidates her experience and individuality
  Discourages her from seeking help

Facts:
  Reactions to rape are varied and individual
  Many women experience a form of shock following a rape that
    leaves them emotionally numb or flat – and apparently calm

Myth: Husbands cannot rape their wives
Implications:
  Assumes that marriage means perpetual consent
  Disempowers married women

Facts:
  It is always rape if the woman does not consent, no matter what
    her relationship with the man

Pickup et al 2001, POWA Information package: gender and violence against women. Online. Available: http://www.powa.co.za/Display.asp?ID=13#myths

the 2001 British Crime Survey established that among women who had been subjected to serious assault including rape since the age of 16, for 52% this led to emotional problems and depression and 5% had attempted suicide.

Early research on domestic abuse failed to recognise the psychological consequences of women experiencing domestic abuse. Paradoxically, whenever the emotional well-being of abused women was being discussed, it was in the context of illuminating how emotional problems would make women more vulnerable to being abused (Gelles & Harrop 1989). More recently, research has dismissed such claims as little more than victim blaming and rightly proclaimed that mental health disorders of domestic abuse victims are an outcome and not a cause of domestic abuse.

Within the UK, there is a growing of body of evidence indicating that the experience of domestic abuse will play a significant role in the development and the exacerbation of mental health disorders, although present day research in this particular area continues to be limited and marginal. Most of the research and evidence in this field originates from studies from the USA, Canada and Australia, where they have correlated domestic violence with adverse mental health outcomes. This includes depression and post-traumatic stress disorder (Cebello et al 2004). In countries such as the USA, Canada, Fiji, Peru, India, Bangladesh and Sri Lanka, suicide is 12 times as likely to have been attempted by a woman who had been abused than one who has not (United Nations 1989).

Post-traumatic stress disorder is a psychological manifestation of a trauma. Learned helplessness is also a condition brought on by violence or more specifically by the inability to stop it (La Violette et al 2000). Domestic abuse and violence are associated with an increased risk for developing a range of psychiatric conditions or intensifying an existing one. At the same time, it could be suggested that living with a mental illness may increase a woman's susceptibility to domestic abuse. Mezey et al (2005) propose it is probable that domestic violence acts as a marker for other traumatic life events that could account for the psychiatric and social difficulties that are often associated to domestic abuse. Studies emerging from the USA have a strong correlation between abuse and mental health.

- Of 140 women attending an out-patient's psychiatric clinic, 64% had a lifetime history of physical and/or sexual abuse (Surrey et al 1990)

- Among 153 women seen in a range of psychiatric settings, over half had been sexually abused and 16% had been physically assaulted as children. As adults, 64% had been sexually assaulted, 36% had been physically attacked and 24% had witnessed severe violence (Mueser et al 1998)
- Out of 303 depressed women, 63% had experienced abuse at some point in their lives; 55% reported having been abused in adulthood by a family member or someone they knew well such as a boyfriend (Scholle et al 1998).

Current available data clearly indicates that women who are being abused by a partner are at increased risk of developing mental health problems such as depression, low self-esteem, post-traumatic stress disorder and suicidal feelings. Studies from the USA and Canada clearly highlighted those women who where receiving services for domestic violence; their rates of depression ranged from 17–72% and for post-traumatic stress disorder 35–88% (Arias & Pape 1999, Humphreys 2003, Humphreys et al 2001, Sackett & Saunders 1999, Street & Arias 2001). Two separate reviews have carried out an analysis of 14 and 17 studies respectively, which clearly identified higher depression rates among abused women: Golding (1999) found an average prevalence rate of 47.6% among abused women and Cascardi et al (1999) exposed depression rates from 38 to 83%.

Abused women have characteristics similar to those of other traumatised populations and they are more likely to exhibit symptoms of post-traumatic stress disorder when they experience high levels of verbal and physical abuse or when they have been victims of forced sex. Psychological and physical abuse is frequently accompanied by sexual abuse in violent relationships. It has been estimated that sexual abuse will occur in 40% of all cases where physical abuse is also occurring. Women who are both physically and sexually abused, are known to have a higher incidence of mental health disturbances than those who experience physical assault alone (Street & Arias 2001). The abuse is often accompanied by other coercive behaviours that may prevent women seeking help. Cascardi et al (1999) suggests that women who experience depression may have been exposed to controlling strategies, which have eroded the woman's sense of self worth. Perpetrators may restrict an abused woman's contact with family and friends while at the same time, limiting her resources to money, enforcing complete isolation on her and reducing her ability to make independent decisions about what she needs (Scholle et al 1998).

In a meta-analysis of US studies Golding (1999) highlighted that the risk of depression and post-traumatic stress disorder associated with partner abuse was even higher than that resulting from childhood sexual assault. Studies have shown that depression in women who are surviving a violent relationship has also been associated with other life stresses that often accompany domestic violence such as childhood abuse. There is also evidence available which demonstrates that the first episode of depression can be triggered by violence and there is longitudinal evidence of depression, lessening with decreasing partner violence (Campbell et al 1997, Campbell & Soeken 1999, Cascardi et al 1999). In a Canadian study, Ratner (1993) discovered that as well as depression, abused women have significantly more anxiety, insomnia and general social dysfunction than non-abused women. It was highlighted that sleep disturbances seemed related to a multifaceted interaction of physical and psychological abuse.

Post-traumatic stress disorder as a consequence of partner violence has also been studied in North America, where it was revealed that the prevalence of depression is much higher in abused women than in non-abused women (Campbell et al 1995, Silva et al 1997). The severity of abuse and partner dominance have been identified as important precursors in post-traumatic stress disorder; suicidal tendencies have also been associated with domestic abuse in the USA and Scandinavia (Golding 1999). Some may argue that marital rape is not a serious crime, and certainly not as serious a crime as stranger rape. However, the evidence does not support this claim; sexually assaulted wives and girlfriends are just as traumatised as women assaulted by a stranger. The after-effects of marital rape are exceptionally destructive and prolonged. Sexually abused women report physical symptoms such as prolonged pain and extreme stress. LaViolette & Barnett (2000) surmise that this may occur because the woman actively inhibits disclosure, feeling that she must hide a shameful secret from close family and friends.

Recognition of the psychological consequences of rape, and the physical symptoms that it creates has led to the term 'Rape Trauma Syndrome', believed to be a form of post-traumatic stress syndrome (Pickup et al 2001).

Studies, which have been carried out in woman's refuges, convenience or volunteer samples of abused women, have indicated that a large percentage, as high as 35–40%, will attempt suicide. Stark & Flitcraft (1995) clearly define that women will attempt suicide because they feel trapped in the relationship and that it is this feeling of entrapment, which may lead women to consider suicide as the only means of escape from her abuser. A retrospective reading of available literature suggests that domestic abuse may be responsible for many women's attempts at suicide. Thus, it is surprising that it has taken so long to make the links between domestic abuse and suicide attempts. Stark & Flitcraft (1995) suggest that female suicide has been influenced by a male bias. While it is true that the typical suicide is committed by a middle-class older white male, the average suicide attempt is made by a younger female who is either married or of a marriageable age, usually between the ages of 33 and 40. Stark & Flitcraft (1995) imply that this profile places characteristics of women at the highest risk for domestic violence, and based on their study, put forward their theory that domestic abuse is a major determinant of female suicide attempts. A harrowing discovery from their study was the realisation that of the women who attempted suicide, over one-third had previously visited the same hospital with an abuse-related injury on the very same day as their suicide attempt. The feeling of 'powerlessness' as described earlier by Stark & Flitcraft (1995) will be increased by the ignorance and barriers that women face from the statutory agencies when they attempt to access help.

The evidence is clear that domestic violence is implicated in one of four female suicide attempts, and features in one-third or more cases of female alcoholism. It is a key factor in drug abuse, female depression and panic attack disorders. Yet mental health professionals are still unlikely to ask about violence during a consultation. Stark & Flitcraft (1996) estimate that as a result of this, less than one case of domestic abuse in ten will be identified.

Childhood abuse and re-victimisation as an adult

Women reporting childhood physical, emotional and sexual abuse have been shown to have an increased vulnerability to physical and psychological abuse as an adult (Coid et al 2001). In particular, childhood abuse has long-term psychological effects, increasing adult vulnerability leading the victims to develop and experience post-traumatic stress symptoms. The likelihood of developing post-traumatic stress syndrome in adulthood is generally increased when the childhood sexual abuse occurred on multiple occasions and was perpetrated by a relative or a significant other person who was held in a position of trust (Briggs & Joyce 1997).

Coid et al (2001) aimed to examine the relationship between childhood trauma and adult re-victimisation. They carried out a cross-sectional survey of 2592 women who were attending primary care practices in east London. Questionnaires were used as their data collection tool. They then analysed associations between childhood and adulthood abuse with multiple logistic regression. The findings of their study demonstrated that childhood abuse substantially increased the risk of re-victimisation in adulthood. Women who had experienced unwelcome sexual intercourse in childhood were more likely to experience other forms of unwanted sexual activity and that the occurrence of either of these also increased their risk of physical abuse as an adult.

In a review of seven North American community-based studies, women who reported a history of childhood sexual abuse also had a significantly higher risk of depression than women who did not report such a history (Weiss et al 1999). This study also demonstrated a two-fold increase in the risk of depression associated with early violent episodes early in life. The risk of depression was highest among those women who had experienced both physical and sexual abuse as a child.

A recent study carried out in the UK by Mezey et al (2005) involving 200 women aged 16 and older and using the maternity services at Guy's and St Thomas' hospital, aimed to estimate the prevalence of domestic violence during pregnancy and following childbirth. A semi-structured questionnaire also included questions about psychological well-being. The Edinburgh Postnatal Depression Scale (EPDS) was used as a data collection tool. Exposure to traumatic events and post-traumatic stress syndrome were measured using the Post-traumatic Diagnostic Scale (PTDS). The study concluded that out of the 200 women who took part in the study, 121 women had experienced at least one traumatic event on the PTDS and 78 of these women had experienced multiple traumatic events. This recent study clearly demonstrates a connection between a history of abuse and current depressive and post-traumatic symptoms. The majority of the women who had endured more than one traumatic event in their lives had higher levels of depressive and post-traumatic stress symptoms than women who had experienced a single trauma. Another important finding of Mezey et al (2005) work was the confirmation that around one in 10 women reported contact with sexual abuse as a child and one in four women had encountered domestic abuse at some point in their lives. Their findings are constant with many UK studies (Council of Europe 2002). Clearly, this work alongside others demonstrates that victims of childhood abuse may have an influence on woman's vulnerability as an adult.

DOMESTIC VIOLENCE AND PREGNANCY

Over the past 20 years, the issue of domestic abuse during pregnancy has received increasing attention, especially in respect to prevalence, effects on the mother and unborn child and whether screening/routine questioning by health professionals should be carried out. However, while this debate continues, it has been realised that domestic abuse is a significant factor in maternal and perinatal morbidity and mortality. The Confidential Enquiry into Maternal and Child Health (CEMACH) (2004) highlighted that 12 women whose deaths were reported to the Enquiry were murdered by their partner. Another 43 women had either voluntarily reported violence to a healthcare professional during the pregnancy or were already known to be in an abusive relationship. These 55 women represented 14% of the women whose deaths were reported to the enquiry. Domestic violence was fatal for 12 of these women. Of the 43 remaining cases, the woman died of other causes. Of the 12 murdered women, 11 were murdered while pregnant or within 6 weeks of delivery. Six of the women were aged less than 18 years and four had been sexually abused in the past. Three of the girls who had suffered sexual abuse were aged 16 years or younger. The CEMACH Report suggests that these figures are probably an underestimation of the true rate of domestic abuse as in none of the 391 cases reported to the Enquiry has a history of violence been actively sought through routine questioning at any point during their pregnancy (CEMACH 2004).

The risk of domestic violence during pregnancy is especially severe, where the health and safety of not one but two victims are placed at risk. Findings from several studies have shown that domestic violence during pregnancy is associated with increased risks of miscarriage, premature birth, low birth weight, fetal injury and even fetal death (Bohn 1990, Stark et al 1979, Webster et al 1996). For almost 30% of women who suffer from domestic abuse in their lifetime, the first incidence will occur during pregnancy (Helton et al 1987, Women & Equality Unit 2004).

Domestic abuse during pregnancy has been linked to repeated miscarriage, antepartum haemorrhage and premature rupture of membranes, premature labour abruptio placenta and intrauterine growth restricted babies (Bullock & McFarlane 1989, Shumway et al 1999, Webster et al 1996). These effects are not ascribed to domestic abuse by many health professionals, they are often attributed to a medical disorder rather than a social disorder and as such remain unchallenged. This may account for the many negative outcomes of pregnancy and birth that remain unexplained.

Abuse in the form of sexual assault and rape can lead to unwanted pregnancies and the dangerous complications that follow in some countries where women resort to illegal abortions (WHO 2002). Women who are in violent relationships are less able to use contraception or be able to negotiate safe sex, therefore they run a high risk of contracting sexually transmitted diseases and HIV and AIDS (Garcia-Moreno & Watts 2000).

The role of the midwife

Victims of domestic abuse will present themselves at healthcare settings with varying physical and mental health problems and if their abuse is identified, they can receive the support and interventions that should improve overall safety and eventually offer an improvement in health and mental well-being. There remains much controversy around routine enquiry and the role of the midwife, and while this debate continues, the health service will continue to deal with the physical consequences of domestic abuse. Several policy and professional documents make clear the role of the health professional in responding to domestic abuse. Asking women about domestic abuse is now becoming accepted as best practice and a professional expectation. The Department of Health has clearly identified the role of the health professional in tackling domestic abuse by stating that public agencies should take every opportunity to identify and support those who are subject to violence (DoH 2005). The recent CEMACH Report (2004) recommends that a routine enquiry should be introduced as standard for all pregnant women, and professional bodies such as the Royal College of Midwives recommends that every midwife assumes a role in the detection and management of domestic abuse (Royal College of Midwives 1999). Yet it is known that clinicians are still unclear about their role in addressing domestic abuse. Many find it difficult to listen to or understand a woman's disclosure and some may even have difficulty in empathising with a victim's powerlessness (Lamberg 2000).

Suggestions for future practice must be that all health professionals should be routinely trained to address and support women who are living in an abusive relationship and likewise domestic violence advocates, professional and voluntary workers, must be prepared to assess the mental health needs of women who are living in abusive relationships. Once that assessment is made, then it is of vital importance that a prompt and appropriate referral is made to the most suitable individual/organisation. The overall lack of national training and partnership working among service providers in the acute and primary care sectors are barriers to optimal care for many women.

A routine enquiry for women's experiences of violence and abuse has to be a key strategy of all health services. There is a wealth of literature available which discusses the benefits of routine enquiry, while recognising that it is not an easy or uncomplicated process. For example, routine questioning in healthcare settings cannot be introduced without adequate training and support mechanisms (Price and Baird 2003, Salmon et al 2004).

CONCLUSION

The physical and psychological consequences of violence against women are immense. However, it is necessary for both medical and therapeutic responses to be coordinated and for any help and support that is offered to women to be available both in the short and long term. The psychological harm caused by domestic abuse may take longer to heal than the physical injuries. Victims and survivors of ongoing psychological and emotional abuse report that living with the emotional torment is often more unbearable than the physical violence.

> 'The body mends soon enough. Only the scars remain . . . But the wounds inflicted upon the soul take much longer to heal. And each time I re-live these moments, they start bleeding all over again. The broken spirit has taken the longest to mend; the damage to the personality the most difficult to overcome'.
>
> (Asia and Pacific Women's Resource Collection Network 1990)

The intertwined relationship between domestic abuse and mental health outcomes should be of interest to every healthcare professional and researcher. Evidence is available that clearly establishes domestic abuse as a major risk factor and cause for many women's physical and mental health problems, the causes and extent of such risks are only recently being realised in the UK. When living with abuse contributes to health factors such as stress, smoking, substance and alcohol abuse and poor nutrition, meaningful interventions to address these coping behaviours will not succeed until domestic abuse is realised and addressed by all agencies at local and Government level.

Research suggests that it is the experience of domestic abuse that actually causes mental health illness in many cases. It must be remembered that the mental health problems of women who are attempting to, or have survived domestic abuse, are the secondary not primary cause of her illness. Clearly, the work of Stark & Flitcraft (1996) around the realisation of domestic abuse and female suicidality, highlights the importance of suicide prevention of routine questioning of all women in healthcare settings following a suicide attempt. Those at specific risk are pregnant women and those women who disclose that a marital quarrel was the precursor of a suicide attempt.

Many studies have shown that women living in violent relationships are restricted in the way they take part in life; in the way they receive love and support from family and friends. They find themselves unable to pursue a job or career. Living in a violent relationship affects a woman's sense of worth and her ability to participate in and enjoy life. Clearly, the overall consequences of domestic abuse are overwhelming, extending beyond the health and happiness of individuals, and affecting the well-being of whole communities (WHO 2002).

References

Amnesty International 1991 Women in the front line. Amnesty international, New York

Amnesty International 2005 Sexual assault research. Summary report. Amnesty International UK. Online. Available: http://www.amnesty.org.uk/images/ul/s/sexual_assault_summary_report_2.doc

Arias I, Pape K T 1999 Psychological abuse: implications for adjustment and commitment to leave violent partners. Violence and Victims 14:55–67

Asia and Pacific Women's Resource Collection Network 1990 Asia and Pacific resource and action series: health. Asia and Pacific Development Centre, Kuala Lumpur

Bohn D K 1990 Domestic violence in pregnancy implications for practice. Journal of Nurse-midwifery 35:86–98

Briggs L, Joyce P R (1997) What determines post-traumatic stress disorder symptomatology for survivors of childhood sexual abuse? Child Abuse and Neglect 21:575–582

Bullock L, McFarlane J 1989 The battering low birth weight connection. American Journal of Nursing 89:1153–1155

Campbell J C, Alford P 1989 The dark consequences of marital rape. American Journal of Nursing 89:946–949

Campbell J C, Belknup R A, Kub J et al 1997 Predictors of depression in battered women. Violence Against Women 3:271–293

Campbell J C, Soeken K 1999 Women's responses to battering over time: an analysis of change. Journal of Interpersonal Violence 14:21–40

Campbell R, Davidson W S, Sullivan C M 1995 Women who use domestic violence shelters: changes in depression over time. Psychology of Women 19:237–255

Cascardi M, O'Leary K D, Schlee K A 1999 Co-occurrence and correlates of posttraumatic stress disorder and major depression in physically abused women. Journal of Family Violence 14:227–250

Cebello R, Castillo M, Caballero G et al 2004 Domestic violence and women's mental health in Chile. Psychology of Women Quarterly 28:298–308

Coid J, Feder G, Petruckevitch A et al 2001 Relationship between childhood sexual and physical abuse and risk of revictimisation in women: a cross-sectional survey. Lancet 358:450–454

Confidential Enquiry into Maternal and Child Health 2004 Improving the health of mothers, babies and children. Why mothers die 2000–2002. RCOG Press, London

Council of Europe 2002 Recommendation of the Committee of Ministers to member states on the protection of women against violence. Adopted on 30 April 2002, with explanatory memorandum. Council of Europe, Strasbourg

Department of Health 2005 Responding to domestic abuse: a handbook for health professionals. HMSO, London

Dobash R E, Dobash R P 1979 Violence against wives. A case against patriarchy. Free Press, New York

Garcia-Moreno C, Watts C 2000 Violence against women: its importance for HIV/AIDS prevention. World Health Organization, Geneva

Gelles R J, Harrop J W 1989 Violence, battering and psychological distress among women. Journal of Interpersonal Violence 4:400–420

Golding J M 1999 Intimate partner violence as a risk factor for mental disorders: a meta analysis. Journal of Family Violence 14:99–132

Heise L 1993 Violence against women: the hidden health burden. World Health Statistics Quarterly 46(1):78–85

Heise L, Ellsberg M, Gottemoeller M 1999 Ending the violence against women. Population reports series, No. 11. John Hopkins University School of Public Health, Population Information Programme, Baltimore

Helton A, Anderson E, McFarlane A 1987 Battered & pregnant: a prevalence study. American Journal of Public Health 77:1337–1339

Hoff L 1990 Battered women as survivors. Routledge, London

Home Office 1999 Domestic violence: findings from a new British crime survey. Home Office Research Studies, London

Humphreys J 2003 Resilience in sheltered battered women. Issues in Mental Health Nursing 24:137–152

Humphreys J, Lee K, Neylan T et al 2001 Psychological and physical distress of sheltered battered women. Health Journal of Psychiatry 144:908–913

James-Hanman D 1999 Domestic violence: breaking the silence. Community Practitioner 71:4040–4047

Kershaw K, Chivite-Matthews N, Thomas C et al 2001 The British crime survey. Home Office, London

Lamberg L 2000 Domestic violence: what to ask, what to do? Journal of the American Medical Association 284:554–556

LaViolette A D, Barnett O L 2000 It could happen to anyone, why battered women stay, 2nd edn. SAGE, London

Lees S 2000 Marital rape and marital murder. In: Hanmer J, Itzin N (eds) Home truths about domestic violence: feminist influences on policy and practice: A Reader. Routledge, London

Mezey G, Bacchus L, Bewley S et al 2005 Domestic violence, lifetime trauma and psychological health of childbearing women. Journal of Obstetrics and Gynaecology 112:197–204

Mooney J 1993 The hidden figure: domestic violence in north London. Middlesex University, London

Mueser K T, Goodman L B, Trumbetta S L et al 1998 Trauma and posttraumatic stress disorder in severe mental illness. Journal of Consulting and Clinical Psychology 66:493–499

Mullen P E, Romans-Clarkson S E, Walton V A et al 1988 Impact of sexual and physical abuse on women's mental health. The Lancet 1:841–845

Pickup F, Sweetman C, Williams S 2001 Ending violence against women. A challenge for development and humanitarian work. Oxfam GB, London

Price S, Baird K 2003 Domestic violence: an audit of professional practice. The Practising Midwife 6:15–18

Ratner P A 1993 The incidence of wife abuse and mental health status in abused wives in Edmonton, Alberta. Canadian Journal of Public Health 84:246–249

Royal College of Midwives 1999 Domestic abuse in pregnancy. Position paper 19a. Royal College of Midwives, London

Sackett L A, Saunders D G 1999 The impact of different forms of psychological abuse on battered women. Violence and Victims 14:105–117

Salmon D, Baird K, Price S et al 2004 An evaluation of the Bristol Pregnancy and Domestic Violence Programme to promote the introduction of routine antenatal enquiry for domestic violence at North Bristol NHS Trust. University of the West of England, Bristol

Scholle S H, Golding J M, Rost K M 1998 Physical abuse among depressed women. Journal of General Internal Medicine 13:607–613

Shumway J, Gielen A, O'Compo P et al 1999 preterm labour, placental abruption and premature rupture of membranes in relation to maternal violence or verbal abuse. Journal of Maternal Fetal Medicine 179:76–80

Silva C, McFarlane J, Soeken K et al 1997 symptoms of post-traumatic stress disorder in abused women in a primary care setting. Journal of Women's Health 6:543–552

Stark E, Flitcraft A 1996 Women at risk: domestic violence and women's health. SAGE, London

Stark E, Flitcraft A, Frazier W 1979 Medicine and patriarchal violence: the social construction of a private event. International Journal of Health Service 9:461–493

Stark E, Flitcraft A 1995 Killing the beast within women. International Journal of Health Services 25:43–64

Street A E, Arias I 2001 Psychological abuse and posttraumatic stress disorder in battered women: examining the roles of shame and guilt. Violence and Victims 16:65–78

Surrey J, Michaels A, Swett C et al 1990 Reported history of physical and sexual abuse and severity of symptomatology in women psychiatric outpatients. American Journal of Orthopsychiatry 60:412–417

United Nations 1989 Violence against women in the family. ST/CSDHA/2. United Nations, New York

Webster J, Battisutta D, Chandler J 1996 Pregnancy outcomes and health care use – the effects of abuse. American Journal of Obstetrics and Gynaecology 174:760–764

Weiss E, Longhurst J G, Mazure C M 1999 Childhood sexual abuse in national survey of adult men and women: prevalence, characteristic, and risk factors. American Journal of Psychiatry 156:816–828

Women & Equality Unit 2004 Domestic violence: key facts. Online. Available: http://www.womenandequalityunit.gov.uk/domestic_violence/key_facts.htm

World Health Organization 1997 Violence against women. WHO Consultation. FRH/WHD/97.8. WHO Geneva

World Health Organization 2002 World report on violence and health. WHO, Geneva

Chapter 10

Suicide and self-harm
Sally Price

INTRODUCTION

Many maternal deaths have traditionally been seen to be physical in origin, such as haemorrhage, sepsis or cardiac disorders. However, within the last reported triennium of 2000–2002, suicide has become the leading cause of the deaths of pregnant women and those who have given birth within the year prior to their death (NICE et al 2004). This is in part due to improvements in methods of data collection and increased identification, but what is particularly shocking is that the majority of these women chose violent methods, including hanging, jumping and intentional road traffic accidents. It is clear that maternal suicide is a significant public health issue, and that the maternity and mental health services should not ignore the mental distress of pregnant and postnatal women. Instead, they should actively seek to provide effective care and support, facilitated by multi-agency collaboration.

This chapter considers the relationship between suicide and self-harm and examines these events in relation to pregnancy and the puerperium. The role of the midwife in identifying women thought to be at risk, along with strategies for effective care will be explored. These factors will be linked to national policy and guidance to provide an insight into how midwives and other healthcare professionals can best support women and their families and promote harm minimisation.

SUICIDE

Rates of suicide vary enormously between countries of origin and gender. For example, the incidence in some former Eastern Block countries is five times higher than in England and Wales, and internationally it is more prevalent in men than women. This has been ascribed to differences in the role of women in society, arrangements for marriage and cultural and religious attitudes to suicide, as well as differences in access to lethal methods for self-harm (NIMHE 2005). There is also a huge stigma associated with death by suicide, particularly in some religious cultures such as Catholicism, where it is considered to be a mortal sin.

Suicide has not been against the law in Great Britain since 1961, although legislation still exists to make it illegal to assist a suicide. In the case of health professionals, the law goes further and it is possible to be sued for negligence in a civil court for failing to safeguard the welfare of a patient or client who proceeds to commit suicide (Taylor & Gilmour 1996). In England and Wales, it is the coroner who decides if a death is to be defined as suicide, based on the evidence of the intent of the deceased. It may be hard to absolutely ascertain the full facts related to the death and a more neutral verdict of open death may be given. Many open deaths are suspected to be suicide and are therefore often considered when determining suicide rates. National data from England demonstrates that there are about 4500 deaths from suicide each year, although the overall death rate has fallen by 6% in recent years. The data also shows that the incidence of suicide varies according to the social group being measured. Although falling to its lowest level for almost 20 years, suicide is most common in younger men (aged 20–34 years), followed by older men and women of all ages (DoH 2005). Suicide during pregnancy is relatively uncommon (NICE et al 2004) with consideration of the baby's needs as a possible protective factor.

Risk factors for suicide in the general population include being single and living alone, being unemployed, having a history of complex mental health problems including self-harm, drug and alcohol abuse, comorbidity and dual diagnoses, being recently discharged from mental health services or non-compliant with treatment regimes and/or disengagement with services (Kirby et al 2004). The methods used also demonstrate some gender differences within the general population. Men are most likely to choose hanging, strangulation or suffocation as a method (46.1%) with less choosing drug-related self-poisoning (18.5%). However, more women choose drug-related self-poisoning (43.9%), often with prescribed psychotropic drugs, with only 25.6% choosing hanging, strangulation or suffocation (DoH 2005). This differs significantly from the maternity population, where 23% of pregnant or postnatal women choosing drug-related self-poisoning to overdose on prescribed medication, and 77% opting for more violent means, such as hanging or jumping (NICE et al 2004) (Table 10.1).

It could be suggested that the choice of violent methods may be linked to the seriousness of the victim's intent. Having access to the means to commit suicide (e.g. firearms) is known to be associated with an increased risk (DoH 2002). However, the link between the act itself and a wish to die may be tenuous, with up to one-third of survivors of a self-harming act reporting feeling ambivalent about whether they died or lived (Hawton et al 1996). What is clear is that there are several factors that are indicative of the intention to die. This includes evidence of pre-planning, with a suicide note and a considered choice of violent method, steps taken to avoid discovery with a conscious isolation of the individual to allow them to undertake the act uninterrupted and regret if failure occurs (DoH 2002, Harrison & Hart 2006).

The risk factors for suicide related to the maternity population appear to differ from the general population. In many of the cases reported to the Confidential Enquiry into Maternal Deaths (CEMACH), health professionals failed to appreciate this (NICE et al 2004). The profile of the 'typical' woman who committed suicide in the 2000–2002 triennium is someone who already has one or more children and is older, married, white and middle class or has a comfortable lifestyle, with a history of previous psychiatric illness and engagement with mental health services and a new baby of less than 3 months old. She is unlikely to have been admitted to

Table 10.1 Methods used for suicide by gender and maternity

	Drug related self poisoning (%)	Hanging, strangulation or suffocation (%)	Jumping or falling (%)	All violent means (%)
Men	18.5	46.1	3.2	49.3
Women	43.9	25.6	4.6	30.2
Pregnant and postnatal women	23	–	–	77

Gender data (DoH 2005). Maternity data (NICE et al 2004).

a specialist mother and baby unit and she is more likely to choose a violent means of death. In terms of the timing of death, women are more likely to commit suicide in the 3 months prior to or the 3 months after the birth of their baby. In some cases, the suicide may also involve the death of an older child or the infant, apart from those babies who die in-utero. However, although rare, most cases of infanticide as a result of serious maternal mental illness are linked to a suicide or suicide attempt on the part of the mother (NICE et al 2004).

The impact of suicide, with or without infanticide must be enormous, particularly on the surviving family members. However, many families live with the mental illness of a relative for many years, and develop coping strategies to deal with this within the family unit. A previous episode of severe mental illness following childbirth gives rise to a 1 in 2–3 chance of recurrence and family members may fail to recognise the seriousness of this or the associated risks of suicide. One case reported to the confidential enquiry demonstrates how the family can support the woman to hide her illness.

> 'There were no concerns about her mental health until the very end of her pregnancy when she called her GP . . . She was diagnosed with agoraphobia and was referred to the community mental health team. She declined psychological intervention on the unusual grounds that the resultant anxiety would harm the baby. This was accepted and no arrangements were made for her to be seen again. Following her death, the family revealed that the woman had wished them to conceal her previous history and that she was developing a paranoid psychosis'.

> (NICE et al 2004:168)

Thus it can be demonstrated that family members may not recognise the severity of a woman's mental illness or anticipate that it could lead to suicide; however, in this case, nor it seems did the clinicians involved in this woman's care. It is evident that health professionals frequently fail to identify risk factors, or if they do, they fail to develop and implement a management plan. The maternity services must be sure to identify those women at increased risk of suicide following birth, and actively seek the collaboration of the woman's family and the relevant support agencies.

A word of caution is necessary at this point. Deaths investigated by the Confidential Enquiry into Maternal Deaths under the category of psychiatric causes of death included several women who died of physical illness such as sepsis. Those providing care misattributed the signs and symptoms of their physical illness to psychological causes, e.g. tachycardia was ascribed to anxiety rather than infection. These findings have resulted in the recommendation that clinicians should remain mindful that 'serious physical illness can co-exist with mental illness. Great caution should be exercised before attributing unusual physical symptoms to psychiatric causes' (NICE et al 2004:169).

SELF-HARM

Self-harm can be viewed as 'an act with non-fatal outcome, in which the individual deliberately initiates a non-habitual behaviour that, without intervention from others, will cause self-harm, or deliberately ingests a substance in excess of the prescribed or generally recognised therapeutic dosage, and which is aimed at realising changes which the subject desired via the actual or expected physical consequences' (World Health Organization, cited by Platt et al 1992).

This definition is complex and possibly unhelpful since it ascribes blame to the individual concerned, particularly by the implication that the act is purposeful, desirable or deliberate. Clearly in some individuals this will be the case, especially if the act is linked to a suicidal intent. However, for many people, self-harming behaviour is not about a wish to die. The meaning of self-harm for the individual involved can vary greatly; for example, it may be as an expression of personal distress or can occur outside the individual's control or awareness (NICE 2004). Self-harm can also be viewed as a coping mechanism or a means to survive previous negative experiences or life situations. This is particularly pertinent to women and pregnancy, with their mental health often rooted in their experiences of violence and abuse (DoH 2003a).

Self-harming behaviour is more likely to occur when people are young, either as a teenager or young adult. It differs from suicide, in that it is more prevalent in women than men. It is also more common in those who lack social support and are socioeconomically disadvantaged. Self-harming behaviour has been linked with those who have a phobic or psychotic illness, and approximately half of all people with a diagnosis of schizophrenia are known to have self-harmed. Many people will receive a diagnosis of mental disorder such as a depression following seeking treatment for self-harming behaviour. There is also an association between self-harm and substance misuse. Some might argue that substance misuse in itself is a form of self-harm but, for example, alcohol is often used as a precursor to a self-harming behaviour such as cutting or poisoning with medication. As well as the above factors, it seems that life events are also of great significance. Those who have lived through severe difficulties or challenging experiences such as sexual abuse as a child, are more likely to adopt self-harming behaviours, and adverse life events such as experiencing domestic violence can be a trigger for acts of self-harm (Kohen 2001).

Case study: ANITA

Consider Anita and her experience of self-harm. At the age of 6, she went into foster care having been removed from her family by social services as a result of being physically abused and neglected by both her parents. She was looked after in several different homes, until a place was found for her with a family who had several other children. At the age of 14, she began running away from her foster parents. It was discovered that a teenage boy within the family was sexually abusing her and she was moved again. By this time, running away had become a way of life for Anita and she was extremely vulnerable, often sleeping rough or with anyone who could put her up. Once she saw a doctor who prescribed antidepressants, but she did not take them because they made her feel sick, and she did not get round to going back. Then she met Mike and felt for the first time that she was with someone who really cared about her. Mike was into drugs and soon Anita was using them too. She began to get into trouble with the police, for minor offences such as theft and prostitution to support their habit, and appeared in court several times. Eventually at the age of 18, she was remanded in custody, prior to being given a prison sentence. As she left court, Mike told Anita that their relationship was over.

In common with other women in the prison, Anita had many of the risk factors that are associated with self-harm. During her life, she had experienced violence within the home, sexual abuse and assault, drug dependency and mental health problems. Experiencing the loss of her relationship with Mike, and being in prison with no social support, triggered Anita's self-harming behaviour of cutting and scratching her legs and arms. When she discovered that she was pregnant, she was quite relieved that the midwife did not mention the marks on her arms when she checked her blood pressure. She continued to self-harm throughout her pregnancy, following the birth of her baby and for the remainder of her sentence.

The method of self-harm that Anita used was cutting, but broadly speaking, the methods people use can be divided in to two groups – poisoning and injury. Poisoning occurs by ingesting a substance harmful to health, usually prescribed or over the counter medicines. Cutting is the most common form of self-injury, but individuals may also stab, shoot, burn and hang themselves. Poisoning appears to be the most common form of self-harming, and is more common in young women (92%) than in young men (84%). The most common poisons used are medicines that can be bought over the counter, such as paracetamol and other analgesics and anti-inflammatory drugs (NICE 2004). However, caution must be used when interpreting statistical data such as this. It is known that those who self-poison are much more likely to seek help, attending venues such as accident and emergency departments (where the data is collected), than those who self-injure. This means self-injury tends to be under-reported as a phenomenon, yet it is more common than self-poisoning among the general population, and particularly among teenagers.

The stigma that is associated with self-harm is huge. The attitudes and behaviour of health service workers who come into contact with people who self-harm have been described as negative, ignorant and punitive (NICE 2004). Often the individuals are blamed for wasting precious health service resources, so it is hardly surprising that many people do not seek treatment or help. However, there can be serious consequences for physical as well as mental health, such as liver failure from paracetamol poisoning. Self-harm can also lead to death from suicide, with a complex association between these types of behaviour.

THE LINKS BETWEEN SUICIDE AND SELF-HARM

The links between suicide and self-harm are complicated and may be confusing to those who are not mental health professionals. There is no doubt that suicide is indicative of acute mental distress and that the risk of suicide is higher in people who have previously self-harmed. However, self-harm may not be based on an intention to die, but as a means to manage mental distress.

Harrison & Hart (2006) propose a useful theoretical model where self-harm is viewed as an over-arching term, with three overlapping, yet separate groups of self-harming motivation and behaviours – communicating or managing negative feelings, impulsive self-harm and attempted suicide.

- Physical self-injury is seen as a means of communicating distress, or managing negative feelings. This may involve feelings of poor self-esteem, anger or frustration and is rarely motivated by suicidal intentions. Typical behaviours include cutting, burning or scratching of the limbs and the individual may be very uncommunicative and withdrawn following the incident
- Impulsive self-harm is often associated with an interpersonal crisis and/or the use of alcohol. Individuals are often ambivalent about dying; simply wishing for the emotional pain to be removed or holding a short-lived perception that death is the answer to their problems. The most common form of self-harm in this group is self-poisoning with medication, and individuals will subsequently seek help following the act, expressing regret or embarrassment at their behaviour
- Third, there are those who attempt suicide. In this case, the individual is unable to contemplate life continuing and has been planning and preparing for the event for several weeks or months. They often use violent means and will have taken measures to ensure they are undiscovered. They are likely to regret that their actions have failed.

Thus, it becomes apparent that for some people, acts of self-harm are separate and distinct from suicide, while for others, both acts are part of the same continuum, with suicide perhaps viewed as the ultimate self-harming behaviour. What is clear is that health professionals should not generalise or make assumptions about the motivation of those they come into contact with. All those who self-harm in any shape or form should be personally assessed and offered care that meets their individual needs.

THE ROLE OF THE MIDWIFE AND OTHER HEALTHCARE PROFESSIONALS

Attitudes and beliefs

The knowledge and skills of all those involved with planning and providing the care for people who self-harm are crucial to the success of any treatment plans. However, equally if not more importantly, so are professional attitudes and beliefs about self-harming and suicidal behaviour. This can be particularly challenging during pregnancy, since both the mother and the baby may be affected by the self-harming behaviour. For example, in simplistic terms it could be suggested that many of us indulge in self-harming activities by smoking cigarettes and drinking too much alcohol. Although these habits are generally becoming less socially accept-able, the woman who smokes or drinks during pregnancy is usually considered negligent and irresponsible by society in general and those who provide maternity care. It could be suggested that con-siderable professional time and energy is spent on cessation pro-grammes that fail to acknowledge the real reasons many women use these drugs of comfort, for example, poverty, desperation and hardship. Women are only too aware that these substances are harmful to themselves and their baby, and most would choose not to use them if there were reasonable alternatives in their lives. However, unless health professionals are able to consider individ-uals holistically, within the context of their own lives and experi-ences, and without prejudice, the care they provide will be of limited value and often fails to meet the woman's needs.

Although these examples may be contentious in relation to the use of the term self-harm, there are some useful parallels between pregnant substance misusers and people receiving treatment for self-harm. Both groups may be shown little respect by their carers. Staff may feel that they are less deserving of treatment than others, which will manifest as poor communication, being rude or curt, and avoiding or keeping the person waiting. The woman is likely to be embarrassed, regretful, or have low self-esteem and experiencing this disrespect may enhance her feelings of shame or guilt. This in turn makes the health professional's task of engaging with the woman much harder and they are both likely to encounter further feelings of negativity. This cycle of blame and shame may reinforce motivation for the self-harming behaviour – the very thing that the health professional should be attempting to alleviate. It is vital that all those working in the health services, including midwives, examine their attitudes and beliefs about self-harm and suicide if they are to be able to offer unbiased and effective care. One way to explore feelings about these difficult issues is to find out and become more knowledgeable about this subject.

Knowledge

Developing knowledge about self-harm and suicide in pregnant and postnatal women is difficult. The majority of research into perinatal mental health has focussed on postnatal depression and puerperal psychosis, as distinct or separate illnesses affecting child-bearing women. The evidence base for effective care of those who self-harm or attempt suicide is scarce, particularly when related to pregnancy and childbirth. There is little published in the professional midwifery press about this subject and practitioners may need to undertake a search of journals outside the sphere of midwifery if they are to find literature that is useful for their clinical practice.

The most useful source of information in the midwifery domain is the CEMACH report (NICE et al 2004) that has identified suicide as the leading cause of maternal death and devotes a chapter to this topic with recommendations for service provision, individual practitioners and education and training (Table 10.2). The 'National Service framework for children, young people and maternity services' (DoH 2004) also makes reference to pre-birth and postnatal mental health needs of women, and confirms the recommendations of NICE et al (2004). Other key documents include more generic information, not specifically related to maternity care. Examples include the 'National suicide prevention strategy for England' (DoH 2002) and 'Mainstreaming gender and women's mental health' (DoH 2003a). Practical guidance on the short-term physical and psychological management of self-harm in primary and secondary care is provided by the 'National clinical practice guideline (16) for self-harm' (NICE 2004).

Becoming familiar with the content of these important policy documents and practice guidelines is a useful starting point for those who work in the field of maternal and perinatal mental health. However, this alone is insufficient. If practice is to be effective, then theoretical knowledge must be applied in the everyday working lives of healthcare professionals. One way to cross the theory practice gap is to work alongside those who have already integrated theory with their practice, and learn from their experience. This means identifying an expert and arranging a placement to spend time shadowing or observing them in practice. Examples might be a community psychiatric nurse with a caseload of perinatal women, a nurse working in a mother and baby unit, or a midwife who is part of a specialist perinatal mental health team. With the changes in the rules around PREP requirements (NMC 2005) this type of professional development has become an acceptable practice, although considerable time management skills are needed to make it possible. An alternative is to reflect on a previous clinical

Table 10.2 Psychiatric deaths from suicide: Key recommendations of the confidential enquiries into maternal deaths 2000–2002

Service provision	Individual practitioners	Education and training
Guidelines for the management of women who are at risk of a relapse or recurrence of a serious mental illness should be in place	Systematic routine enquiries about previous psychiatric history, its severity, care received and clinical presentation should be made at the antenatal booking visit	The Royal Colleges of Psychiatry, Obstetrics and Gynaecology, General Practice and Midwives should ensure that perinatal psychiatry is included in their curricula and requirements for continuing professional development
A specialist perinatal mental health team should be available to provide care for those at risk or suffering from serious postpartum mental illness	All relevant information about the woman's previous or current psychiatric history should be included in their referral letters to the booking clinic	
Postnatal women who require psychiatric admission should be cared for in the nearest specialist mother and baby unit along with their baby	The term postnatal depression or 'PND' should not be used as a generic term for all types of psychiatric disorder. Details of the illness should be sought and recorded	Local training must be put into place before routine screening for serious mental illness is implemented
Sufficient regional psychiatric mother and baby units should be developed to meet the needs of the population	Women with a history of serious psychiatric disorder should be assessed by a psychiatrist in the antenatal period, and a management plan agreed and recorded in case of a recurrence	Obstetricians and midwives should be aware of the laws and issues that relate to child protection and when and to whom to refer if concerned
	Women who have previously experienced a serious mental illness at any point should be counselled about the risk of recurrence following pregnancy	

(NICE et al 2004).

experience and consider how the practice could have been improved in the light of new knowledge. Other learning activities may include becoming familiar with local and national voluntary and statutory services that are available to support women who experience mental illness, not only during the perinatal period, but also at any point in their lives. This may provide another avenue in which to identify 'experts' who can help develop practice, and be useful in ensuring clients receive the on-going support they need.

Developing skills

Having attended to the physical effects or injuries, many non-mental health trained professionals doubt their ability to provide further effective care for those who self-harm or attempt suicide. Common reasons for not engaging with the client include feeling afraid of the individual and their own feelings, not wanting to make the situation worse and uncertainty about the treatment and support available to those who self-harm. However, developing the skills to provide effective care is not insurmountable. Indeed many of the skills required will already be well developed in experienced healthcare workers such as empathy, listening, observation and evaluation. Professional confidence can be developed through exploration of attitudes and beliefs via appropriate training, and enhanced through increased knowledge and the support of supervisors of midwives and peer groups.

Effective communication is at the core of any interaction between professional and patient, and this is essential in the case of self-harm or suicide. From openness and honesty, trust can develop, empowering the client to identify their needs and participate in the planning of their care. However, to identifying the care needs of someone who presents with an injury from self-harm or attempted suicide, it is essential to undertake a risk assessment of recurrence. In most cases, this should be undertaken by a trained mental health professional. However, the reality is that this may not be possible due to the management of resources, or the client not being prepared to wait, particularly if their injuries do not warrant admission to hospital. Unfortunately, there are no validated tools to assist the non-mental health practitioner, and none seem to be targeted for pregnancy and the postnatal period. However, this does not mean that midwives and other healthcare workers should do nothing and refer the 'problem' to the mental health services. Indeed, there is a professional responsibility for all health service workers to ensure that they care for those with mental health needs in a holistic and safe manner (DoH 2003b). Without a risk assessment, it is impossible to argue that the individual is safe or has been cared for in an appropriate way.

In practical terms, a risk assessment is not impossible for the non-mental healthcare professional to undertake. What is important is for the limitations to be recognised with appropriate follow-up planned and provided by the mental health team. The key factors when undertaking this type of assessment are to determine the risk of serious harm or death occurring in the short term. Known risk factors from the evidence base such as NICE et al (2004) can be useful, although not every woman who attempts suicide will fit the criteria. Observing the individual and considering if they are anxious, withdrawn, inattentive, aggressive or behaving inappropriately, can be useful. Exploration of the antecedents of the event and the woman's access to immediate and on-going social support should also be undertaken. Consideration should also be given to child protection issues. Health professionals should share their concerns with women in a non-threatening way to ensure children are not exposed to avoidable risks. This may include recognising the needs of the whole family, involving them as well as the woman in risk assessment, care planning and provision. Other community-based practitioners can make a useful contribution with the woman's consent, such as GPs, health visitors and religious ministers, where appropriate.

A crucial factor in risk assessment is establishing a meaningful dialogue with the woman. Listening to what she says about her feelings and actions may be most insightful, since it is important to remember that for some women, self-harm is not about wanting to die, but allowing themselves to express emotions they would otherwise find intolerable (Suyemoto 1998). In this type of situation, using a 'harm minimisation' approach may be helpful (Box 10.1) and demonstrates respect for the woman's autonomy and right to self-determination. However, if effective communication cannot be established, the woman's needs may best be met by the specialist mental health team.

CONCLUSION

Suicide and self-harm are serious public health issues. Prevention and harm minimisation should concern all health workers, not just those who are mental-health trained. Being pregnant or having

Box 10.1   A harm minimisation approach

Health professionals should aim to:

- Adopt a non-judgemental attitude to understand the reasons why women self-harm, based on listening to what they say
- Provide the means for individuals to retain their autonomy, dignity and responsibility as far as possible
- Actively support and encourage women to take steps to contain their self- harming behaviour within reasonable limits, and work with them to replace self-harming with more positive user-led coping mechanisms
- Provide a means by which women can address the underlying causes of their self-harm
- Advise and support women to take care of their own injuries unless urgent medical treatment is required
- Clarify the circumstances in which staff have a responsibility to protect, that overrides the individual's autonomy, e.g. when the self-harm is life-threatening, even if without intent
- Recognise their own and others need for support when providing care for women who self-harm.

(DoH 2003a)

recently given birth does not necessarily protect women from these events, with suicide as the leading cause of maternal death. While in need of improvement, the evidence base provides information on risk factors, and national guidance is available to support practice. Health workers, especially midwives, need to develop the knowledge and skills of risk assessment to provide effective primary care prior to referral to specialist mental health services. It is essential that all those who come into professional contact with people who have self-harming behaviours display genuine empathy and understanding, with non-judgemental attitudes. Without this, any attempt to plan and provide care in partnership with the client will fail.

References

Department of Health 2005 National suicide prevention strategy for England. Annual report on progress 2004. DoH, London

Department of Health 2004 National service framework for children, young people and maternity services. DoH, London

Department of Health 2003a Mainstreaming gender and women's mental health. DoH, London

Department of Health 2003b Essence of care. Patient focused benchmarks for clinical governance. DoH, London

Department of Health 2002 National suicide prevention strategy for England. DoH, London

Harrison A, Hart C 2006 Mental health care for nurses: Applying mental health skills in the general hospital. Blackwell Science, Oxford

Hawton K, Ware C, Kingsbury S 1996 Paracetamol self-poisoning characteristics, prevention and harm reduction. British Journal of Psychiatry 168:43–48

Kirby S, Hart D, Cross D et al 2004 Mental health nursing. Palgrave MacMillan, Basingstoke

Kohen D 2001 Psychiatric services for women. Advanced Psychiatric Treatment 7:328–334

National Institute for Clinical Excellence 2004 Self-harm: The short term physical and psychological management and secondary prevention of self-harm in primary and secondary care. National clinical practice guideline, No. 16. NICE/British Psychological Institute and the Royal College of Psychiatrists London

National Institute for Clinical Excellence, The Scottish Executive Health Department, and The Department of Health Social Services and Public Safety: Northern Ireland 2004 The confidential enquires into maternal deaths in the United Kingdom. Why mothers die 2000–2002. NICE/RCOG Press, London

National Institute for Mental Health in England 2005 International variations in suicide rates. National Electronic Library for Health. Online. Available: www.kc.nimhe.org.uk

Nursing and Midwifery Council 2005 The PREP handbook. NMC, London

Platt S, Bille-Brahe U, Kerkhof A et al 1992 Parasuicide in Europe: the WHO/EURO multi-centre study on parasuicide. 1. Introduction and preliminary analysis for 1989. Acta Psychiatrica Scandinavica 85:97–104

Suyemoto K 1998 The functions of self-mutilation. Clinical Psychology Review 18:531–554

Taylor S, Gilmour A 1996 Towards understanding suicide. In: Heller T, Reynolds J, Gomm R et al (eds) Mental health matters. Palgrave MacMillan, Basingstoke

Chapter **11**

Who cares for the carer? Support for the midwife

Rosemary Mander

INTRODUCTION

The relationship between the woman and the midwife is fundamental to midwifery care. In some circumstances, such as emergencies, this relationship may need to develop very quickly. In
normal situations, the relationship matures over the duration of the
woman's pregnancy, resulting in a confident and trusting relationship by the time it is most needed – during the labour and the birth.
If this relationship is fundamental to women with an 'uncomplicated' pregnancy, how much more important is it to the woman
who has experienced or is experiencing mental health problems?

This chapter argues that the midwife *is* able, through this relationship, to provide effective support for the woman with mental
health difficulties. In order to demonstrate the strategies by which
the midwife establishes the relationship with the woman, the development of this relationship is reviewed. If the midwife is to provide
good support, she should in turn be able to locate and utilise her
own support system. Hence, this chapter examines some of the
skills and resources on which the midwife may draw. In this way,
the ideal of the well-supported midwife offering effective support
to the woman emerges. Attention is also given here to those situations in which this pattern may prove to be not only idyllic, but also
mythological.

Although this may not always apply to midwives working in the
National Health Service, the assumption is made here that some
element of continuity features in the woman's care. So the relationship which is discussed below is one which endures for a period
of months, and possibly years, rather than the one which extends
only over a matter of hours or days. It is necessary to bear in mind

the huge variation in the organisation of maternity care, even in a country the size of the UK.

This chapter differs from the others in this book in that it is written in the first person. Although some may regard this as informal or 'chatty', I make no apology for this form. The rationale is that, whereas in the other chapters, the emphasis is on the woman who is the consumer or recipient of care, in this chapter the emphasis is on the midwife, who is the care provider. This form serves to remind us all that midwives are not invulnerable to the mental health problems which are the focus of this book.

BUILDING THE RELATIONSHIP

The relationship between the woman and the midwife ordinarily begins with what is still known as the 'booking' or the 'booking interview'. It is possible, however, that there may have been prior acquaintance, possibly during a previous pregnancy or, in the case of the independent midwife, during an initial meeting for the woman and midwife to decide whether a formal booking was appropriate.

It is during the booking interview that the foundations of the relationship are laid. The orientation towards childbirth education is clarified, as is the use of research evidence by both the woman and the midwife. Thus, the level of participation in decision-making becomes understood. Whereas much of what is written about the booking interview focuses on the form-filling and record-making, Methven (1990:49) extends this 'information-gathering exercise' as far as the woman's physical assessment and examination and the necessary investigations. The groundwork of the relationship, which Methven (1990:49) actually goes on to refer to as a 'partnership', is established at this interview, which includes the preliminary moves in balancing the roles and relative power of the two major participants.

The tendency of midwives to under-utilise the relationship-enhancing opportunities presented by the booking interview is well recognised. In her research which, admittedly, was undertaken nearly two decades ago, Methven (1990) found that the midwives who did not work in the antenatal clinic on a long-term basis deliberately avoided entering into a relationship with or engaging with the woman. The disconcerting corollary to these midwives' reluctance is found in the behaviour of the 'permanent' midwives; they, while clearly recognising the significance of the booking interview, regarded their role as being a more administrative one to ensure the smooth running of the clinic and 'keeping an eye on the doctors' (Methven 1990:61). It is to be hoped that this example of midwives' adherence to the medical model is now less noticeable. Unfortunately, I have not been able to identify any material to show that this is the case.

Maternal history taking

Much of the literature on the booking interview relates to the content, in terms of the topics to be addressed and areas covered. A crucial component of the booking interview is the taking of the maternal history (NHS QIS 2004). Some attention, however, has been given to the communication skills necessary to obtain accurate information as well as laying the foundations of the interpersonal relationship. In their account, Gask & Usherwood (2002) achieve a balance between these major aspects of such an interview with an admirable emphasis on the appropriate use of communication skills. It is these skills which will develop and then maintain the interpersonal relationship which may serve as supportive to the woman with mental health problems. Gask & Usherwood show the need for the member of staff to observe all the usual 'social niceties', such as being welcoming, providing introductions and using the name with which the client is comfortable. As with so many activities, it may be useful to think of the booking interview in terms of the beginning, the middle and the end; the application of which may be summarised as 'say what you're going to do, do it and then say what you've done'. In this way, the woman should find the meeting not only non-threatening, but also helpful.

Communication

The two main modes of communication in the context of the booking interview, as in many other situations, are verbal communication and body language or non-verbal communication. In referring to the latter, O'Driscoll (1997) summarises the activities according to the level of learning required. These activities range from the 'rapid eye-brow-flash' (O'Driscoll 1997:422), which is universal and probably totally intuitive, to gestures such as the 'double thumbs up', which invariably need to be learned. The use of body language has recently attracted considerable attention from a range of occupational and professional groups in relation to emotion work or emotional labour. These activities feature the ability, as part of one's work, to create an acceptable ambience or successful outcome, by hiding one's real feelings (Hochschild 1983). This topic is now beginning to be given the attention which it deserves in relation to midwifery and childbearing (Hunter 2004).

It is difficult, if not impossible, to clearly separate non-verbal from verbal communication. This problem becomes most easily apparent in the use of active listening. This technique involves the listener, by the use of both non-verbal and verbal cues, in making the process of communication an active or two-way phenomenon. As well as adopting an interested posture and nodding and vocalising appropriately, the active listener will maintain a comfortable level of eye contact; although what constitutes comfortable is largely determined by the culture in which the interaction is happening. Further, the active listener will summarise what she understands the speaker to have said and will reflect back what the speaker has been saying, which may comprise content or perhaps emotions. In this way, feelings of empathy become more firmly established between the two participants.

The verbal content comprises what the listener does not say as much as what she does say. The dangers of interrupting the speaker are many (Gask & Usherwood 2002), especially because interruptions are likely to deter the speaker from confiding any further. Even if left to speak unconstrained, the speaker is not likely to continue for more than 1 min.

In building a relationship, it is crucial to notice and to respond to the cues which the woman offers. Like interruptions, failure to act on these 'openings' deters the speaker from creating any more. These skills are extensions of the active listening mentioned already. In order to prompt or to stimulate such 'openings', the listener should avoid the 'closed' questions, which can be answered with just a single word. 'Open-ended' or 'non-directive' questions require that the speaker, observing the social conventions of conversation, is obliged to respond more expansively. In her observational research on midwives' conducting booking interviews, Methven (1989) reports that non-directive questions were notable by their absence. On those rare occasions when the midwives used them, their encouraging effect was countermanded by a closed question being interjected before the woman had time to answer.

The professional approach

Sometimes for a midwife, establishing a relationship with a child-bearing woman is less than straightforward. This is partly because there may be difficulties in deciding where to draw the line between being the professional healthcare provider and being the woman's friend. This difficulty should come as no surprise, bearing in mind the virtual universality of the experience of childbearing. This difficulty may cause problems for the midwife however, who is uncomfortable about sharing, or not sharing, such a ubiquitous experience. Under such circumstances, the term 'professional' assumes an unusual, perhaps even a slightly perverse meaning. This is because it serves to demarcate or provide an artificial barrier between two people with much in common who are working towards a common goal. 'Professional' here is unrelated to the quality of the service or the care, but merely to the creation of psychological distance, lack of engagement and even some kind of hierarchical relationship between the two participants. This issue emerged in my own research (Mander 2006) on the care of the woman who does not have her baby with her, because the baby may have died, or is in the neonatal unit or is being relinquished for adoption. The midwives recounted to me their thoughts about whether it is correct for the midwife to share the tears of the bereaved woman. For one of the midwives, her reluctance came down to issues of 'professionalism':

> Bessie: There are really two schools of thought about [staff crying]. First, there is the old school which says that you must retain your professional thing quite intact. The second view is that you grieve with the woman. I think that it really depends on the midwife and the woman. I am quite happy to hold her hand or to put my arm round her shoulder, but I think that you need to stay a professional.

Other midwives were equally aware of the debate, but were confident that crying was not unhelpful and may actually be beneficial:

> Emily: I know some people think that it is not professional, but I do sometimes cry with the mother as this lets her see that we are human.

> Ottily: You can have a little cry . . . and nobody thinks any the less of you. You never used to be able to do that.

Ticking boxes

The caring relationship with the woman may occasionally be undertaken by more than one care provider. In such circumstances, effective communication between the carers is essential. This is one of the few situations, I would argue, when the use of checklists is actually beneficial. Unfortunately, possibly due to the increasingly litigious nature of maternity care, or perhaps because litigation fears have been imported from across the Atlantic, checklists are being used far more frequently. This approach to care not only jeopardises any individualisation of care and impedes communication, it also reduces care to the lowest common denominator. That checklists are used as often as they are is an unfortunate reflection on midwifery in the UK healthcare system.

A notable exception to this critique of the use of checklists is found in a study undertaken in England by McCabe (2004). She sought to facilitate communication between people with severe and enduring mental health problems and their carers. Both patients and their medical care providers reported that the quality of communication was improved by the use of checklists. This was apparent in the increased length of the interaction by an average of 13 min. Thus, in this setting, the use of checklists actually appears to have served to facilitate communication, rather than the reverse.

Family involvement

In the valuable analysis of history taking by Gask & Usherwood (2002), probably appropriately, they consider the role of family members in the interaction with the healthcare provider. These authors emphasise the need to acknowledge the family member's presence and to include him in the interaction. Interestingly and without explaining their rationale, they suggest that if the patient is an adolescent who is accompanied by a parent, part of the interview should be held without the adult being present.

In maternity care, the involvement of the baby's father is often regarded as a welcome development in the care of the childbearing woman (Mander 2004a). It is widely argued that the involvement of the father in the pregnancy and the birth lays the foundations for healthier and more satisfying father–child relationships. This involvement is likely to include not just supporting the woman when she attends for her antenatal checks and assisting with her care during the labour and birth, but may also include providing support for her and getting to know the baby in the postnatal ward.

The point at which a partner's presence may cease to be supportive and starts to become oppressive may be difficult to judge. But midwives have begun to take note of those occasions when the father shows signs of becoming just that bit too attentive, because this may be associated with domestic violence (Mezey 2002). The need for the midwife to be able to speak to the woman without her partner being present has resulted in the use of a range of novel strategies, which permit the woman and midwife 'confidential time' (Mezey & Bewley 2000). For this reason there should be time made available, at least during the booking interview, when the male partner is not present. Whether it is feasible to obtain this confidential time at booking and whether the midwife is able to use it to the woman's advantage is quite a different matter. It may be more likely that the woman will be less anxious about taking the midwife into her confidence when their relationship is better established.

Women's experiences

The woman's impressions of the development of the relationship between her and the midwife emerged serendipitously in a study of flexible antenatal care (Sanders 2000). Some of the women in this RCT were disappointed at the delay before the first contact with the midwife:

> *Having found out quite early that I was pregnant, it seemed a long time before I was booked in to see the midwife. Even though my doctor was lovely and told me the food I shouldn't be eating, I came away thinking 'Oh – is that it?' I appreciate that there isn't much that can be said or done in early pregnancy, but I found out more information from buying a pregnancy book and reading magazines.*
>
> *(Sanders 2000:171)*

Other women, regardless of their parity, reported the value they attributed to their developing relationships. One woman mentioned how highly she valued the reassurance provided and:

> *To know that someone is constantly aware of you and your baby's health.*
> *(Sanders 2000:172)*

The more analytical qualitative study by Edwards (2000) focussed on the experiences of a group of women who were planning to give birth at home. Some of the women were quite clear about the high standard they expected of their relationships with the midwife:

> *There won't be fear in the air, there'll be a sort of expectation, yeh, we can do this together.*
> *(Edwards 2000:68)*

Edwards found, though, that the women's experiences of forming a relationship with the midwife varied considerably. Perhaps as a result of their high expectations, some of the women were seriously disappointed:

> *It's like you're bombarded with things that you don't want and not getting the things you do want.*
>
> *(Edwards 2000:68)*

One woman was so disillusioned that she felt impelled to change her booking in order to achieve the relationship which she sought. She reported on the later, successful relationship:

> *The difference . . . is because I have time to get to know her [the midwife], as what normally happens is that she comes round, we have a cup of tea, we have a chat . . . then by the time she's been there for 45 minutes or an hour we do the check, so she will do all these things, but it seems relevant; it's like someone you know who's caring for you, checking that you're okay, so it feels different that you're not straight in the door and on the scales or straight in the door and lying on your back with your top up; you've actually engaged as an adult with somebody first.*
>
> *(Edwards 2000:68)*

In spite of some women's serious disappointments, Edwards' work shows that for a few women, their high expectations of the relationship developing with the midwife may prove to be satisfied:

> *There came a stage when I really wanted her to be absolutely with me, I just remember looking really hard into her eyes and she absolutely meeting that stare, and taking it in and giving me strength just through the way she looked at me, which is exactly what I needed.*
>
> *(Edwards 2000:69)*

Assessing social support

As this study by Edwards' (2000) demonstrates, there is a possibility that the relationship between the woman and the midwife may prove to be supportive precisely when the woman needs that support. That the support of the midwife can be effective is significant for the woman for a number of reasons. In the present context, the established link between lack of support and mental health problems endorses the importance of the relationship with the midwife (SIGN 2002). In order to operationalise this research evidence, a quantitative research project was undertaken in Brisbane, Australia to validate an instrument measuring the extent of the woman's social support (Webster et al 2000). The researchers anticipated that the six-item instrument would be able to be applied routinely when the woman is seen for her booking interview.

Webster and her colleagues inevitably found that some of the women scored low on the instrument. They interpreted this to mean that the woman was poorly supported. Such assumed lack of support was found to be significantly associated with a collection of factors. These included the woman booking later, experiencing poorer general health both pre- and postnatally, making more frequent contacts for medical attention and showing a greater likelihood of developing postnatal depression. The sensitivity of this Australian instrument, though, is open to question. There remains a suspicion that this six-item questionnaire did little more than identify a cohort of women whose lives featured a range of problems, of which a lack of support and mental health difficulties were but two.

A more general question about this Australian study, though, relates to the ethics of assessing social support. If the researchers had been successful in their aim of identifying poorly supported women, what intervention would have been made in order to remedy the situation? Does the Australian healthcare system have the resolve or the resources to provide effective support for these vulnerable women in order to prevent the occurrence of their mental health problems? If not, this study is unethically misleading to those who are involved.

In response to this criticism, it may be helpful to mention the community action approach by midwives in the relatively deprived Cowgate district in Newcastle upon Tyne. This project clearly demonstrated how social support may be provided effectively (Davies 1997, 1990, Evans 1997). Unfortunately, for the present context, the intervention was evaluated largely in terms of perinatal health, rather than maternal health.

The challenges

Up to this point in this chapter, I have been considering the challenges which the midwife may encounter when seeking to develop a relationship with a childbearing woman. These challenges apply irrespective of the health or 'normality' of the woman's childbearing experience, but I venture to suggest that these challenges are exacerbated or aggravated if the woman's childbearing experience deviates from the mythological standard textbook model of normality. Such deviation includes the woman who develops or is experiencing mental health difficulties. In these circumstances, the midwife is likely to find that she is, through her relationship with the woman, providing supportive care with the aim of facilitating the woman's return to optimal functioning and preventing any harm to the woman and/or to her baby.

It may be that developing and maintaining such a supportive relationship may be regarded as 'all in a day's work' for the midwife. It is necessary to question, though, whether it is reasonable to expect midwifery staff to provide such a high level of emotional commitment, which verges on the psychotherapeutic relationship. If the answer to that question is 'Yes', then for how long is such an input possible, before it begins to take its toll and the personal costs become too great for the midwife to bear? And what form do those personal costs take? In the next section, I consider the costs which the midwife may have to pay and the risks to which she is vulnerable.

THE PERSONAL COSTS TO THE MIDWIFE

Having examined, in the first section, the challenges facing the midwife in establishing and maintaining relationships which are supportive to her women clients, I now consider the costs to her personally. These costs may be levied on her as a midwife, on her as a family member or on her as a woman.

General costs

In order to consider the wide range of effects on the midwife in her multiplicity of domestic and professional roles, I consider first the more general effects of these challenges. I then gradually focus down on to the more precisely mental health-related issues. I have found that there is a dearth of material in the literature relating to the midwife and mental health issues. For this reason it is necessary, here and throughout this chapter, for me to apply material from other areas to the role and the experience of the midwife.

Stress

The costs and challenges which I have mentioned already may manifest themselves in the form of stress. The term 'stress', however, fails to make the crucial distinction between negative and positive stress. The type of stress which I am considering here is that to which this term is most commonly applied, that is, the negative form of stress.

Particularly relevant here is the work by Munro et al (1998) which focussed on Australian psychiatric nurses to examine negative forms of occupational stress. These authors refer to Karasek's distinction between job strain and occupational stress. Strain is regarded as the more negative phenomenon because, in the presence of high stress or psychologically demanding work, the individual has little control over their own activities. Thus, there is unresolved conflict with which the person must also cope. The symptoms of this outcome would include fatigue, anxiety, depression and the risk of physical illness. On the other hand, if the job's demands are high and the individual has a high level of control over their work, Karasek (1989) maintains that the rewards are correspondingly great. Thus, although the job continues to be stressful, this constitutes a positive form of stress.

In the study by Munro and colleagues, a five-part questionnaire was applied to 100 nurses and obtained a commendable 60% response rate. The areas addressed by the questionnaire included health, job satisfaction, job control, job demand and social support. This research endorsed the relevance of the model proposed by Karasek. It went on to show, however, that teamworking offered higher levels of job demands, but at the same time provided greater job control than traditional hierarchical structures. This research is useful because it illuminates the different forms of stress which people working in the mental health field may encounter.

Burnout

Like 'stress', burnout has attracted considerable attention, not all of it entirely justified:

> [Burnout] has become the helping professions' equivalent to what the British army called 'shell shock' or the Americans 'battle fatigue'; what our parents' generation called 'nerves' and the present generation 'depression'. They become catch-all phrases that signify not coping.
>
> (Hawkins & Shohet 1989:20)

The significance of burnout in the 'helping professions' is related largely to the professionals' unrealistically high expectations of their own ability and invulnerability. While they, through their work, are acutely aware of their clients' weaknesses, they are blind to or ignorant of their own human frailty. The crucial difference between 'stress' and 'burnout' may be found in the time span of the two conditions. Whereas stress is an acute condition, typically occurring in response to an incident or an event known as a stressor, burnout is more of a process, happening over a longer timeframe. Burnout, while initially a psychological process to produce outward affective and physical symptoms eventually involves the worker's negative experience of job strain and results in this characteristically maladaptive form of psychological adjustment.

The phases of burnout are summarised in the traditional definition offered by Burnard:

'A syndrome of emotional exhaustion, depersonalization and reduced personal accomplishment'.

(Burnard 1991)

The midwife's burnout has attracted particular attention through two important studies. The first is the Dutch study by Bakker et al (1996). These researchers focussed on 200 community midwives and their work. Data were collected through detailed diaries, one questionnaire on practice and personal characteristics and another questionnaire on burnout, coping and social support. The researchers found that the midwife's degree of depersonalisation correlates positively with the size of the group practice within which she works, rather than with the level of urbanisation of her working environment (Bakker et al 1996:180). They also found that a higher proportion of home births is associated with a lower risk of burnout which, the researchers suggest, is likely to be mediated by greater job satisfaction. The corollary of this observation is that a high proportion of short-stay hospital admissions relates more to profound emotional tension.

The other major study on the midwife's burnout was undertaken in England by Sandall (1997, 1998, 1999) using a mixed methods research design. Sandall showed that that autonomy, social support and meaningfulness of relationships with women were significant themes. All of the midwives valued collegial social support as a stress reducer. When such support was lacking, however, this lack itself constituted a major source of stress. The midwife's domestic support or lack of it was found to have similar effects. The presence of children may be perceived as either a stressor or as a buffer against stress, but Sandall found that children serve to prevent the midwife embarking on unhealthy over-commitment to her work. Similarly, children may actually prevent the midwife from becoming involved in certain over-taxing practice arrangements.

Approximately one-fifth of the midwives claimed to be burned-out in association with a lack of collegial support, fragmented client contact, too heavy a workload, too high expectations, or lack of domestic emotional/social support. On the other hand, the midwives with high levels of personal accomplishment reported assertive and realistic relationships with colleagues, women and 'family', collegial work support, domestic emotional/social support, meaningful client relationships, appropriate non-work time and non-work activities. Sandall was able to draw conclusions about certain organisational structures' links with burnout.

Sandall argues, on the basis of her findings, that burnout should be re-defined in terms of disillusionment, rather than the three characteristics mentioned above.

Distancing

One of the classic signs of burnout has been labelled 'depersonalisation' (see traditional definition above). This behaviour is characterised by the carer's detachment leading to alienation from both clients or patients, and from colleagues. Negative feelings about those with whom she works are prevalent to the extent that avoidance tactics may be employed, such as becoming immersed in mindless administrative tasks.

This pattern of coping clearly resonates with the classic work by Isobel Menzies (1960). In this groundbreaking study, Menzies identified the difficulty encountered by nurses in facing the impact of forming relationships with and providing care for sick and dying people in hospital. Menzies went on to analyse the routines, rituals, structures and hierarchies which had been developed as crucial to providing care in such an institution. Many of these activities would fit into the 'mindless' category mentioned above. These strategies served as defence or coping mechanisms, to limit engagement with patients. In this way, they could be used to protect nurses from potentially painful interactions with those for whom they were caring.

The strategies recognised by Menzies, which are also characteristic of burnout, are disconcertingly similar to the 'professional' attitudes and behaviour mentioned previously.

Bullying

The phenomenon which is known as bullying, 'mobbing' or horizontal violence' may be another example of the price which the midwife may find herself having to pay for the challenges of the relationships which she develops (Mander 2004b). As mentioned already, a characteristic feature of burnout is the lowering of self-esteem. This reduced self image, in turn, predisposes to the bullying behaviour with which we are all likely to be familiar. At an organisational or inter-professional level, horizontal violence may make its presence known through similar manifestations. In this situation, the members of an oppressed group begin to assail their peers in a variety of ways. This happens because the oppressed group is impotent to contend with the major oppressor who threatens all of them. Thus, what manifests itself is a form of aggression against equals who, for some reason, are not in a position to defend themselves (Field 2002).

Impairment and attrition

The costs of forming meaningful relationships, to which I have been referring, are essentially costs to the midwife herself. It is necessary to bear in mind, though, that through her impaired functioning, these costs may be levied on the maternity service of which she is a part. In this way, the costs may need to be shared by the midwife's colleagues and subordinates and even by the women for whom she provides care. In this way, the costs of her engagement may be spread both widely and indiscriminately.

Another cost which the midwife may be required to meet is that which takes the form of her changing her practice. This is an outcome which emerged in a recent research project (Mander 2005). Although New Zealand midwives have passionately embraced the opportunity there to practice autonomously as lead maternity carers (LMCs), the negative stress which they encounter in that role is causing a disconcertingly large number to move out of independent practice into hospital midwifery employment. It may be that this move is temporary, constituting a 'revolving door' of midwifery practice.

A more severe form of such changing practice could be found in the midwife abandoning midwifery practice completely. This outcome is a tragedy. For a midwife who engages conscientiously and effectively with her women clients, to relinquish her practice as a direct result of her conscientiousness and effectiveness is nothing less than an abysmal reflection on her working conditions. I consider below, the action which may be taken to prevent this tragic outcome.

Costs related to mental health issues

After considering the costs of engagement which may apply both generally and in the care of women with mental health problems, I now focus on certain problems which may be particularly associated with a range of personnel working in mental health care. Many of the costs mentioned have already been shown to feature prominently in the field of mental health. This statement derives from the work of Goodwin & Gore (2000), which involved the observation of interactions between staff and clients in a long-stay residential care facility in England. These researchers found that, as Menzies demonstrated in 1960, social distancing was often used to protect the staff from engagement. This was achieved by activities limiting the humanity of the clients, such as by discussing a client's need for new underclothes in a public setting (Goodwin & Gore 2000:318). Goodwin & Gore also identified the strategy used by staff to cope with their own feelings of vulnerability and dependency. In order to do this, the staff minimised the differences between themselves and the clients, through jokes and games, through sharing decisions and through role reversal (Goodwin & Gore 2000:320). Goodwin & Gore also refer to the observation of reduced contact time with clients being associated with higher levels of burnout. These researchers conclude that the culture of reluctance to engage, which Menzies found half a century ago among nurses in an acute setting, is still prevalent in a long-term mental health service. There is no reason to believe that nurses are unique, or that people working in such a setting are unique.

Identification

The inclination of the general public to differentiate themselves from people with mental health problems by regarding them as 'not like me' may constitute a defence mechanism. However, there is a tendency among health workers to identify with those for whom they care, which may manifest itself in a variety of ways. This tendency appears in comments which often relate to what the health-care worker would do or not do if they found themselves in a particular situation. How many times have we heard colleagues reflect on: 'If it was me, I would . . .' or 'I wouldn't . . .'?

Such identification featured in the midwives' comments during my research project on the care of the woman who does not have her baby with her, because the baby may have died, or is in the neonatal unit or is being relinquished for adoption. When discussing the contact the woman might or might not have with, for example, her stillborn baby, one midwife clearly tried to put herself into the woman's place, by telling me:

> I certainly would not want to cuddle anything that was dead myself.
> (Mander 2000:34)

In a more recent project, on the midwife's experience of providing care for a woman who dies (Mander 2004c), similar feelings of identification were reported to me by a midwife with some pastoral responsibilities:

> ... as [the midwives] were in the same age group as the mother they readily saw themselves in the same situation.
> (Mander 2004c:44)

Because some of the midwives were in a different age group, their feelings of identification were less directly with the woman who died:

> This is partly because my own daughter is the same age as she was. I feel that if she ever gets pregnant I'll be one worried person (nervous laugh).
> (Mander 2004c:44).

Such problems with identification tend not to feature prominently in the midwifery literature. They have, however, been recognised in cancer nursing (von Klitzing 1999), as well as in disaster situations, where they have been shown to engender 'a high degree of distress' (Ursano & McCarroll 1995:56). Identification has been shown, in a review of the literature on nurses working in disaster situations, to constitute an important component of nurses' responses (Robbins 1999).

Personal boundary maintenance

The latter, rather extreme examples may serve to clarify the costs which the midwife working with women with mental health problems may be required to pay. The existence of personal boundaries is well recognised in those areas of care which may involve an element of counselling or psychotherapy (Marshall 2001). As well as the obvious physical boundaries, they may take an emotional, relational, spiritual or sexual form. They are built around what is safe and appropriate for the client and practitioner. Marshall defines boundaries in terms of 'flexible and inflexible limits that let good in and keep bad out' (Marshall 2001:3).

Ordinarily, boundaries are comfortable and healthy, but under certain circumstances, problems may arise, as mentioned above. Thus, boundaries may become excessively rigid, to the point of acting as defences, or they may even be damaged. Of particular concern is when boundaries are violated. This may happen inadvertently and we have all learned from such embarrassing errors. More disconcerting are the deliberate violations, which may happen when the violator has some form of power over the violated. Examples might include adult/child, employer/employee and even professional/client relationships. The bullying mentioned above might be an example of such a violation.

Those who care for people with mental health problems are particularly likely to encounter problems in appropriately maintaining the integrity of their personal boundaries. Henderson (2004) suggests that these problems are associated with the 'caring' relationship having the potential to transform itself through the use of mental health legislation. In this way, the facilitating role or 'power to' is converted into the invariably paternalistic 'power over' (Dowding 1996).

Transference

Another phenomenon which is said to be 'universal' (O'Kelly 1998:392) may also bring with it implications, and perhaps costs, for the midwife (Green 2005). This is 'transference', which is an unconscious process involving the displacement of behaviours, thoughts and feelings from their original context; they are transferred on to another person, possibly someone in a caring role. Transference is not necessarily a negative process, as it may bring with it strong feelings of affection or admiration. However, feelings of hatred or anxiety may be introduced into the new relationship through transference. These reactions are likely to be stimulated by a temporary situation in which the person feels worried, frustrated or traumatised (O'Kelly 1998:392).

The relationship between the woman and the midwife would be fertile ground for the occurrence of transference towards the midwife. The likelihood of this happening may be exacerbated if the woman feels vulnerable due to mental health problems.

In psychotherapeutic settings, O'Kelly maintains that the therapist works hard to become anonymous, in the hope that transference will not limit the effectiveness of the therapy. For the midwife, however, such anonymity is not feasible due to the relationship being more equal, even being widely regarded as a partnership

(Pairman 2000). For this reason, the midwife may find herself becoming the object of the transference of a variety of emotions.

Dependency

In her relationship with a woman demonstrating a serious degree of transference, the midwife may find that the woman is effectively becoming addicted to her and the care which she provides. This is likely to result in the woman becoming excessively dependent on the midwife and in her being unable to complete the psychological and other tasks which are fundamental to pregnancy and new motherhood. Dependency is a feature of mental health problems, with the client being at risk of becoming dependent on agents such as the medication, the health services or, as is of concern in the present context, the person who provides care (Ryan 1998).

The costs

It is apparent that even in the care of the healthy childbearing woman, there may be personal costs which the midwife may need to take into account. When she is providing care for a woman with mental health problems, a further range of costs may be superimposed on those ordinarily present. It is inevitable that, while these costs are being exacted of the midwife, they will also impinge to a greater or lesser extent on those close to her. Thus, her partner and family may also find themselves feeling the impact of her work-related challenges. So, too, will the colleagues alongside whom she works. These costs may be comparable with the 'coping deficit' identified by Lazarus & Folkman (1984), when the individual perceives the demands of the situation as exceeding her coping abilities.

I will now examine the strategies which may be implemented by the individual, by the peer group and by the employing organisation (if any) to ensure that the personal costs to the midwife do not become too excessive.

POTENTIAL REMEDIES – SUPPORTING THE MIDWIFE

I have already considered the role of the midwife in building and sustaining caring and supportive relationships with her childbearing clients. What has also emerged are the personal costs to her, in her various roles, and to those who are near to her. I now examine the possible remedies available to the midwife, which may facili-

---

Box 11.1   Alleviation of stress: some suggested strategies

Organisational

- Clinical supervision
- Employee assistance programmes
- Family activity
- Peer support
- Reflective practice
- Self care
- Statutory supervision
- Supportive practice
- Teamworking
- Time management.

Personal/individual

- Autogenic regulation training
- Counselling
- Cultivating assertiveness
- Exercise
- Journalling
- Massage
- Medication
- Progressive relaxation
- Relaxation with desensitisation
- Stress inoculation training
- Substance use
- Yoga/meditation.

(Some strategies from Bailey & Clarke 1989)

---

tate her effective functioning while minimising the personal costs. These remedies manifest themselves in a variety of forms. They happen at different levels, involve different personnel, have different organisational input and extend over different time periods (Box 11.1).

The multi-professional or multidisciplinary team

Teamworking, rather like leadership, may be presented as something of a panacea. Teams, in this context including occupational therapists and community psychiatric nurses, may be regarded as the solution to a wide range of organisational and other difficulties, such as overstressed personnel. The reality of teamworking, however, may be something different again and requires close examination (McCallin 2001:420).

The uncertain benefits of even single professional teamworking were demonstrated in the research on community nurses by Griffiths & Luker as long ago as 1994. An immensely strong organisational culture was identified, in which intraprofessional conflict was to be avoided at all costs in order to give a semblance of mutual support and harmony within the team. The price of this 'teamworking', however, was found to be a serious reduction in patient choice and, more importantly, a seriously compromised quality of care.

More recently, using a case-study approach, Freeman et al (2000) found that when it proved effective, teamworking was perceived as being immensely supportive to the members of the multiprofessional team. Unfortunately, though, the team members' differing interpretations of the meaning of being a team member meant that such effective teamwork was not easily achievable. These authors observe that these differing interpretations threatened communication and understanding of each others' roles. For this reason, underlying resentments could be exacerbated, professional esteem could be undermined and 'outright conflict' could actually be created (Freeman et al 2000:238). Thus, the supportive nature of teamworking has been called into question.

The many overlapping features of team activity and leadership may be assumed to mean that these two organisational phenomena may be equally overrated. There is a possibility, though, that leadership may have benefited from the mass of attention which it has received. The result is that effective leadership may provide better support for personnel experiencing excessive levels of negative stress. The work of Eagly & Carli (2003) is particularly relevant in the present context, as they argue that the increasing numbers of women in leadership roles means that more human and humane leadership styles are gaining precedence. By this, these authors mean that transformational leadership styles, which adopt a more 'shared vision' approach to achieving goals, are more successful when used by and among women. This is in comparison with the more macho transactional approaches which tend to appeal to subordinates' self interest, rather than team or service user benefits.

Supportive practice

Useful insights into the effectiveness of providing 'top down' support in practice situations is provided using a psychotherapeutic orientation by Playle & Mullarkey (1998). These authors draw comparisons between the ways in which practitioners care for the client and the way in which they care for each other. They refer to these comparisons as 'parallel processes'. Although these writers draw on the relationships characteristic of their mental health background, their argument is more than relevant to midwifery, especially if the support of the midwife caring for a woman with mental health problems features. The nub of Playle & Mullarkey's argument is that if a staff member is to provide effective care by engaging appropriately with the woman or client, then that member of staff must be confident of having an effective, supportive and open relationship with a mentor, preceptor or supervisor. In this way, the hopefully therapeutic relationship of the childbearing woman with the midwife who attends her is comparable with or parallels the hopefully similarly healthy and supportive relationship of the midwife with her own supervisor.

Self care

The argument that the midwife should be able to find effective support if she is to provide effective support, should not diminish the possibility of the midwife obtaining support for its own sake. Kirkman (2001) takes a welcome common sense approach to the benefits of the midwife adopting strategies to care for her own mental health in spite, rather than because, of the multiplicity of challenges which she faces. These strategies include locating sources of support and asking for help when it is needed. Kirkman offers us a refreshing reminder of our own and others' humanity, albeit with all the associated weaknesses.

Peer support

The negative stress associated with working in an emotionally challenging setting is widely thought to be alleviated by interaction with colleagues. This assumption was investigated in an acute mental health setting by a quantitative study involving 93 qualified and unqualified nursing staff (Jenkins & Elliott 2004). These researchers found that the support of fellow workers was directly beneficial in reducing levels of emotional exhaustion. The importance of this support was attributed to the unique understanding of colleagues and their being 'on the spot'. Other potentially supportive people, such as a supervisor or family member, were considered less supportive due to their not being available to the same extent.

The findings of Jenkins & Elliott's study (2004) resonate with the findings of my qualitative study of the midwife's experience of caring for a woman who dies (Mander 2004c). This group of seriously traumatised midwives told me of the sources of support which they found to be effective. The support which was generally found to be most valuable was, like in the acute mental health setting, that offered by colleagues. Those who were most helpful, though, were colleagues with either the same or a similar experience. As one midwife told me:

> *The ones who are most understanding are those who were actually there that night or at least those who were on duty at the time. I find that things have changed. It is my colleagues who were really good and I have become close to the other midwives who were on with me that night and who shared the experience. Before that, they were just the people I worked with but now they have become my friends. I feel we have a lot in common and I have become close to them.*

> *Midwife 20*

For some of the midwives, though, others who were not actually involved were not regarded as supportive:

> *. . . everybody who was actually involved in the incident was very, very supportive and really helped me a lot and was coming round to see me when I was off sick. Y'know being very, very nice and at that time I didn't feel I could talk to an outsider about it. I wanted to talk to people who knew her [the woman] like I knew her. The midwife who looked after her for the 2–3 days before I met her – and I wanted to be with people who knew the situation rather than with people who didn't know and I felt wouldn't understand.*

> *Midwife 12*

Thus, the effectiveness of peer support was clearly variable.

Alternative sources of support

In my study of the death of a mother, the family also emerged as important sources of support to the midwives:

And fortunately, a lot of us had good partners so we had good support at home.

Midwife 8

... my husband. I don't need him to say anything, I just need him to listen to me. That's how I cope. He does not have to say anything. He does not need to comment, may be he'll just say that's awful or something like that. That's all I need. Some people say that their pets are like that – someone to talk to.

Midwife 7

Oh I batter my poor old husband to death. Verbally [laughing]. His solution to everything 'cos he's a chef is to create me something tasty. Laugh.

Midwife 17

This tendency to find support in her domestic life may be a characteristic of a woman's coping (Etzion 1984). This applies in comparison with the more male dominated setting where Jenkins & Elliott (2004) undertook their research. Etzion argues that men invariably find their support network among their colleagues. This support may happen in the workplace or in a relaxing setting after work. For women, though, these 'relaxing settings' may be less appropriate because of family obligations.

Reflective practice and professional education

Long before it was hailed as an educational instrument, reflection was being recommended as a therapeutic tool by both Freudian psychoanalysts and behaviourists (Mantzoukas & Jasper 2004). Since the ground-breaking work of Schon (1983), however, the importance of reflection has been extended to benefit not only the practitioner, but also her practice (Johns 1995). Reflection-in-practice, followed by reflection-on-practice serve to move the practitioner's learning from the factual into the realms of experiential learning. In this way, a virtuous cycle of learning begins to escalate. Inevitably during this cycle, her self-awareness develops exponentially, bringing with it opportunities to revisit and rework stressful experiences. In this way, improved self-knowledge facilitates more effective ways of handling and coping with challenging situations. In many pre-registration, as well as post-registration programmes, reflective and experiential learning are becoming increasingly important as they serve to build on the learner's previous life experience.

Clinical supervision

Since its introduction, clinical supervision has been intended to ensure the emotional health of the practitioner, as well as ensuring the development of effective relationships with clients. Playle & Mullarkey (1998) trace the development of this form of support from those disciplines which are accustomed to employing psychotherapeutic approaches. Subsequently, clinical supervision has been used in closely related disciplines, such as counselling and social work and then by disciplines related to them such as mental health nursing and learning disability nursing.

The definition of what constitutes clinical supervision varies. The managerial input is a particular source of concern as, ideally, it should be non-existent. The supervisorial relationship may be described in terms of protecting clients, or therapy, or education or a combination of all three. In their authoritative paper, Playle & Mullarkey (1998) regard clinical supervision as comprising elements of support, education and management; but they admit that the balance between these elements varies. While the literature emphasises support and education, practice tends to focus more on the management or 'quality control' aspects which serve to protect the client, especially since the significance of clinical supervision was emphasised by the Allitt Enquiry (Clothier 1994).

Clinical supervision has assumed greater importance because more holistic approaches to care and more equal relationships between clients and carers have limited the possibility of traditional defence mechanisms, such as distancing (Menzies 1960). Such 'partnerships' have additionally created new challenges to care providers, such as transference and blurring of boundaries.

Compared with the purely mental health fields, midwifery has only relatively recently become interested in clinical supervision (Deery 2005). The community-based action research project which Deery implemented, sought to address some of the organisational challenges facing the midwife at the beginning of the twenty-first century. Of prime concern among these challenges is the inexorably changing working environment. For Deery the increasingly equal relationship between the woman and the midwife is seen, not as a partnership (see Pairman 2000), but as a threat of 'new powers and more influence' (Deery 2005:162).

Unlike Playle & Mullarkey (1998), Deery defines clinical supervision almost entirely in terms of its psychosocial benefits to the supervisee, namely support and enabling. The support deficits which became apparent in Deery's action research project included managerial and financial support as well as team support. She concludes that her limited success in introducing clinical supervision to a team of community midwives is attributable to the midwives' inadequate knowledge of group dynamics. To this deficiency, she also adds their need to develop 'interpersonal skills at a high level' (Deery 2005:173).

Statutory supervision in midwifery

Midwifery supervision derives from the inspection of midwives which was introduced in England with the Midwives Act of 1902 (Stapleton et al 1998). It is unsurprising, therefore, that it developed into a managerial form of supervision, sometimes known as 'snoopervision'. The traditional aim, however, has been to protect the public by ensuring safe standards of midwifery practice (Duerden 2002). The role of the supervisor of midwives is determined by the Midwives Rules, through which she is delegated the responsibility of ensuring that the midwife reaches and maintains a satisfactory level of competence. Isherwood (1988) describes this difficult role in terms of offering support by being a 'guide, counsellor and friend' to the midwife over whom she also happens to have the power to suspend from duty and perhaps from practice (Isherwood 1988:65).

An authoritative research project (Stapleton et al 1998) has further served to investigate the imbalance between the emphases on supervisor as 'watchdog' or as 'friend', to which Isherwood (1988) refers. This project, commissioned by the English National Board and the UKCC, comprised, first of all, an audit of supervisors and arrangements for supervision. The second, qualitative, part of the project involved in-depth interviews and focus groups with midwives, with supervisors and with users of the midwifery services. Following the collection of these data, midwives provided their personal constructs which allowed a value grid to be drawn up. The data were collected at five contrasting sites in England. The sixth 'site' comprised midwives whose practice was outwith the mainstream NHS maternity care system.

This research project found that, first, the existence of unhealthy power relationships leads to the stereotyping and blaming of clients. In this way, not only is the inverse care law (Stapleton et al 1998:32) brought into effect, but the spectre of horizontal violence also materialises (Stapleton et al 1998:21). The second major finding was the midwife's awareness of the need for support. This applied to both the woman and the midwife, but was in marked contrast to the reality of the lack of any support for either. The third finding related to the dearth of suitable role models; this could be exacerbated by an ineffective form of supervisorial support, which extended to the point where the midwife was providing support for the supervisor. The fourth and final finding was the unhealthy culture of the social environment in which the midwife practises. Its unhealthy nature is related to the longstanding emphasis on the midwife coping remorselessly with whatever happens and conforming to the organisational stereotype.

As a result of this fundamentally important research project, changes have been implemented in the organisation of midwifery supervision. Some midwives consider that the situation has been corrected (Rodger 2004). Other midwives, on the other hand, consider that statutory midwifery supervision still lies at the root of the problem of midwives' lack of autonomy (O'Connor 2002).

CONCLUSION

In this chapter, I have attempted to outline the nature of the challenge facing the midwife caring for the woman with a mental health problem. I traced the development of the crucial relationship which the midwife needs to forge with the woman. This led to consideration of the price which the midwife, and those near to her, may have to pay for maintaining this relationship. Finally, I reviewed the remedies which the midwife may access to alleviate the stress which she encounters in what may be a difficult relationship.

The conclusion which emerges is that for the midwife who invests her well-being in order to engage with a woman with mental health problems, there is little organisational backing. This midwife all too often must fall back on her own resources – her family and her equally stressed colleagues.

Acknowledgement

I would like to thank Fiona Boswell for her help in the preparation of this chapter.

References

Bailey R, Clarke M 1989 Stress and coping in nursing. Chapman & Hall, London

Bakker R H C, Groenewegen P P, Jabaaij L 1996 'Burnout' among Dutch midwives. Midwifery 12:174–181

Burnard P 1991 Coping with stress in the health professions: a practical guide. Chapman & Hall, London

Clothier C M 1994 The Allitt Inquiry: independent inquiry relating to deaths and injuries on the children's ward at Grantham and Kesteven General Hospital during the period February to April 1991. HMSO, London

Davies J 1990 Against the odds. Nursing Times 86:29–31

Davies J 1997 The Newcastle community midwifery care project: The evaluation of the project. In: Thomson AM, Robinson S (eds) Midwives Research and Childbirth, Vol. 2. Chapman & Hall, London, p 115–140

Deery R 2005 An action-research study exploring midwives' support needs and the affect of group clinical supervision. Midwifery 21(2):161–176

Dowding K 1996 Power. Open University Press, Buckingham

Duerden J 2002 Midwifery supervision. In: Mander R, Fleming V (eds) Failure to progress: The contraction of the midwifery profession. Routledge, London

Eagly A H, Carli L L 2003 The female leadership advantage: An evaluation of the evidence. The Leadership Quarterly 14:807–834

Edwards N P 2000 Women planning home births: their own views on their relationships with midwives. In: Kirkham M (ed.) The midwife-mother relationship. Macmillan, London, p 55–91

Etzion D 1984 Moderating effect of social support on the stress burnout relationship. Journal of Applied Psychology 69:615–622

Evans F 1997 The Newcastle community midwifery care project: the project in action. In: Thomson A M, Robinson S (eds) Midwives research and childbirth, Vol 2. Chapman & Hall, London, p 104–114

Field T 2002 Times Educational Supplement, 21.06.02.

Freeman M, Miller C, Ross N 2000 The impact of individual philosophies of teamworking on multiprofessional practice and the implications for education. Journal of International Professional Care 14:237–247

Gask L, Usherwood T 2002 ABC of psychological medicine. The consultation. British Medical Journal 324:1567–1569

Goodwin A M, Gore V 2000 Managing the stresses of nursing people with severe and enduring mental illness: A psychodynamic observation study of a long-stay psychiatric ward. British Journal of Medical Psychology 73:311–325

Green A 2005 Personal communication

Griffiths J M, Luker K A 1994 Intraprofessional teamwork in district nursing: in whose interest? Journal of Advanced Nursing 20(6):1038–1045

Hawkins P, Shohet R 1989 Supervision in the helping profession: an individual, group and organizational approach. Open University Press, Buckingham

Henderson J 2004 Continuing professional development. The challenge of relationship boundaries in mental health. Nursing Management (London) 11:28–32

Hochschild A R 1983 The managed heart: commercialization of human feeling. University of California Press, Berkeley

Hunter B 2004 Conflicting ideologies as a source of emotion work in midwifery. Midwifery 20:261–272

Isherwood K 1988 Midwives' Journal. Friend or watchdog? Nursing Times 84(24):65

Jenkins R, Elliott P 2004 Stressors, burnout and social support: nurses in acute mental health settings. Journal of Advanced Nursing 48:622–631

Johns C 1995 Framing learning through reflection within Carper's fundamental ways of knowing. Journal of Advanced Nursing 22:226–234

Karasek R 1989 Control in the workplace and its health-related aspects. In: Sauter S, Hurrell JJ, Cooper CL (eds) Job control and worker health. John Wiley, New York, p 29–59

Kirkman S 2001 How to . . . preserve your mental health. MIDIRS Midwifery Digest 11:432

Lazarus R S, Folkman S 1984 Stress, appraisal and coping. Springer, New York

Mander R 2000 Perinatal grief: understanding the bereaved and their carers. In: Alexander J, Levy V, Roth C (eds) Midwifery practice: core topics 3. Macmillan, London, p 29–50

Mander R 2004a Men and maternity. Routledge, London

Mander R 2004b The B-word in midwifery. MIDIRS Midwifery Digest 14:320–322

Mander R 2004c When the professional gets personal – the midwife's experience of the death of a mother. Evidence based Midwifery 2:40–45

Mander R 2005 Perceptions of decision-making in relation to maternity care organisation and place of birth in New Zealand and Finland. Unpublished report

Mander R 2006 Loss and bereavement in childbearing, 2nd edn. Routledge, London

Mantzoukas S, Jasper M A 2004 Reflective practice and daily ward reality: a covert power game. Journal of Clinical Nursing 13:925–933

Marshall A 2001 Oops, you're stepping on my boundaries! NATCON Papers. Canada. Online. Available: http://www.contactpoint.ca/resources/dbase.php?type=user_query&fetched=1149

McCabe R 2004 Checklist improves communication between doctors and patients and results in changes in care. Evidence Based Mental Health 7(3):86

McCallin A 2001 Interdisciplinary practice – a matter of teamwork: an integrated literature review. Journal of Clinical Nursing 10:419–428

Menzies I E P 1969 (1960) A case study in the functioning of social systems as a defence against anxiety. In: MacGure J (ed.) Threshold to nursing. Bell, London

Methven R 1989 Recording an obstetric history or relating to a pregnant woman? A study of the antenatal booking interview. In: Robinson S, Thomson AM (eds) Midwives research and childbirth, Vol 1. Chapman & Hall, London

Methven R 1990 The antenatal booking interview. In: Alexander J, Levy V, Roch S (eds) Midwifery practice: antenatal care: a research-based approach. Macmillan, London, p 42–57

Mezey G C 2002 Domestic violence. Report CR102. Royal College of Psychiatrists Council

Mezey G C, Bewley S 2000 An exploration of the prevalence and effects of domestic violence in pregnancy. ESRC. Online. Available: http://www.regard.ac.uk/research_findings/L133251043/report.pdf 16 August 2002

Munro L, Rodwell J, Harding L 1998 Assessing occupational stress in psychiatric nurses using the full job strain model: the value of social support to nurses. International Journal of Nursing Studies 35:339–345

NHS Quality Improvement Scotland 2004 Best practice statement: maternal history taking. NHS QIS, Edinburgh

O'Connor M 2002 'Good girls' or autonomous professionals? Part III: beyond statutory supervision: quality assurance and the equality agenda. MIDIRS Midwifery Digest 12:159–164

O'Driscoll M 1997 Interpersonal skills. In: Henderson C, Jones K (eds) Essential midwifery. Mosby, London, p 421–440

O'Kelly G 1998 Countertransference in the nurse-patient relationship: a review of the literature. Journal of Advanced Nursing 28:391–397

Pairman S 2000 Women-centred midwifery: partnerships or professional friendships. In: Kirkham M (ed.) The midwife-mother relationship. Macmillan, London, p 207–226

Playle J F, Mullarkey K 1998 Parallel process in clinical supervision: enhancing learning and providing support. Nurse Education Today 18:558–566

Robbins I 1999 The psychological impact of working in emergencies and the role of debriefing. Journal of Clinical Nursing 8:263–268

Rodger M 2004 The supervisor of midwives' role in protecting the public: a focus in the arena of public health. MIDIRS Midwifery Digest 14:541–545

Ryan T 1998 Perceived risks associated with mental illness: beyond homicide and suicide. Social Science Medicine 46:287–297

Sandall J 1997 Midwives' burnout and continuity of care. British Journal of Midwifery 5:106–111

Sandall J 1998 Occupational burnout in midwives: new ways of working and the relationship between organizational factors and psychological health and wellbeing. Risk Decision and Policy 3:213–232

Sandall J 1999 Team midwifery and burnout in midwives in the UK: practical lessons from a national study. MIDIRS Midwifery Digest 9:147–152

Sanders J 2000 Let's start at the very beginning . . . Women's comments on early pregnancy care. MIDIRS Midwifery Digest 10:169–173

Schon D 1983 The reflective practitioner. Avebury, Aldershot

Scottish Intercollegiate Guidelines Network 2002 Postnatal depression and puerperal psychosis: a national clinical guideline. SIGN, Edinburgh

Stapleton H, Duerden J, Kirkham M 1998 Evaluation of the impact of supervision of midwives on professional practice and the quality of midwifery care. University of Sheffield and ENB, Sheffield

Ursano R J, McCarroll J E 1995 Exposure to traumatic death: the nature of the stressor. In: Ursano R J, McCaughey B G, Fullerton C S (eds) Individual and community responses to trauma and disaster. Cambridge University Press, Cambridge, Ch 3

von Klitzing W 1999 Evaluation of reflective learning in a psychodynamic group of nurses caring for terminally ill patients. Journal of Advanced Nursing 30:1213–1221

Webster J, Linnane J W J, Dibley L M et al 2000 Measuring social support in pregnancy: can it be simple and meaningful? Birth 27:97–103

Chapter **12**

Mental health, mental illness and pregnancy

Sally Price

This book has covered a wide range of topics related to mental health, mental illness and pregnancy. It has also considered how midwives and other health professionals can best serve the women they care for. The authors are from diverse backgrounds yet have each used their own experience and expertise to examine how mental health, mental illness and pregnancy are interlinked. This is perhaps the most valuable aspect of the book, enabling readers to consider their own philosophy and approach to care. However, it becomes clear that supporting women with mental health disorders requires a diverse approach and is not the domain of any one professional group. All too often mental health or rather, mental illness is seen as a speciality that is outside the role or boundaries of professional groups other than those within the psychiatric services. This is perhaps due to a lack of awareness or understanding of mental illness and approaches to care, but may also be due to the fear, stigma and stereotyping of mental illness. The maternity service, and those who work with pregnant and postnatal women must get to grips with this field of work, and ensure that women receive the care they need and want.

However, it is also vital that midwives and the maternity services acknowledge the mental healthcare needs of their predominantly female profession. They are exposed to the same social and physiological risk factors as the women they care for, with the additional stresses of their working lives. Self care is essential, but they should also be able to expect the support of peers, managers and supervisors of midwives. Care and regard for each other's mental health is sometimes sadly lacking within the midwifery profession. Midwives need to feel valued and respected to promote their mental well-being. If they are unable as a professional group, as midwifery teams and as individuals to support each other in this way, then they cannot hope to meet the needs of their service users.

Promoting mental health, treating mental disorders and supporting women and their families is not easy, although this book gives a summary of the evidence related to different successful approaches such as medication, talking therapies and social support. The authors have also given a raft of information about the practical skills and interventions that can support practice. Many of these suggestions are evidence-based tools that can be used simply and easily. Other ideas and concepts provide practitioners with the foundations to build upon and identify their own specific learning needs. Equipped with this knowledge, it is hoped that practitioners will work effectively to benefit service users, and meet their needs, however complex. What is certain is that no one profession or service can tackle this alone. Harrison & Hart (2006) identify that effective perinatal mental healthcare is dependent upon collaboration and interdisciplinary working between and within healthcare teams, in particular effective liaison and joint working between primary healthcare, secondary mental healthcare and the maternity services. Supporting women with mental health disorders can never be a single agency issue and the maternity services and mental health service must operate collaboratively. If this is achieved, then perhaps the tragedy of suicide as the leading cause of maternal death can be avoided.

Reference

Harrison A, Hart C (eds) 2006 Mental healthcare for nurses: applying mental health skills in the general hospital. Blackwell, Oxford

Appendix

Useful websites

Centre for Evidence-based Mental Health	www.cebmh.com
Depression Alliance	www.depressionalliance.org
Disability Rights Commission	www.drc-gb.org
Mad Pride	www.ctono.freeserve.co.uk
Mental Health Foundation	www.mentalhealth.org.uk
Mental Health Matters	www.mental-health-matters.com
Mind	www.mind.org.uk
National Institute of Mental Health	www.nimh.nih.gov
National Institute for Mental Health in England	www.nimhe.csip.org.uk
Refuge	www.refuge.org.uk
Rethink	www.rethink.org
Royal College of Psychiatrists	www.rcpsych.ac.uk
Sainsbury Centre for Mental Health	www.scmh.org.uk
Samaritans	www.samaritans.org.uk
Sane	www.sane.org.uk
Social Exclusion Unit	www.socialexclusion.gov.uk
Young people and self harm	www.selfharmuk.org
Victim Support	www.victimsupport.org
Women's Aid	www.womensaid.org.uk

Index